CBT for Hoarding Disorder

CBT for Hoarding Disorder

A Group Therapy Program Workbook

David F. Tolin
Bethany M. Wootton
Blaise L. Worden
Christina M. Gilliam

WILEY Blackwell

This edition first published 2017
© 2017 John Wiley & Sons Ltd

The right of David F. Tolin, Bethany M. Wootton, Blaise L. Worden, and Christina M. Gilliamto be identified as the authors of this work has been asserted in accordance with law.

Registered Offices
John Wiley & Sons, Inc., 111 River Street, Hoboken, NJ 07030, USA
John Wiley & Sons Ltd, The Atrium, Southern Gate, Chichester, West Sussex, PO19 8SQ, UK

Editorial Office
The Atrium, Southern Gate, Chichester, West Sussex, PO19 8SQ, UK

For details of our global editorial offices, customer services, and more information about Wiley products visit us at www.wiley.com.

Wiley also publishes its books in a variety of electronic formats and by print-on-demand. Some content that appears in standard print versions of this book may not be available in other formats.

Library of Congress Cataloging-in-Publication data applied for

ISBN Paperback: 9781119159247

Cover Design and Illustration: Wiley

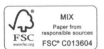

Contents

Chapter 1/16

Welcome to the Class

1. Welcome to the Declutter Class

Welcome to the Declutter Class! We are glad to have you on board.

The Declutter Class is designed to be a 16-week class with each class lasting for 90 minutes. This workbook will provide you with the information you need to learn and practice the skills from the Declutter Class. We encourage you to complete all of your treatment assignments directly in this workbook. You will see that there are

CBT for Hoarding Disorder: A Group Therapy Program Workbook, First Edition. David F. Tolin, Bethany M. Wootton, Blaise L. Worden, and Christina M. Gilliam.

spaces to write in throughout the workbook. This document contains much of the same information that your class leaders will talk to you about during the class.

Here are a few important things about the class and this manual:

1. **Class tasks**:   During the class we will be teaching you lots of new information and skills. We will also do lots of tasks together while we practice discarding and resisting acquiring. When you see this picture of a group discussion it means that we will do a task together as a class. These tasks will vary, but they are an important part of the class.

2. **Rita's story**:   When you see the image of the woman on the right it means that this part of the manual is "Rita's Story." Rita will explain how she used the skills in order to overcome her problem with clutter. You will see her story whenever you see her picture. You can follow her story across the 16 weeks of the class.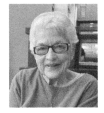

3. **Sorting and discarding**:   The goal of this class is to help you to reduce your clutter. We'll do this by having you practice sorting your possessions by putting them into different boxes. Our experience shows us that people in the class do best when they practice sorting and discarding using three boxes:

   a.   Keep
   b.   Donate/Recycle
   c.   Trash

   We will be using this system throughout the class and we will practice sorting and discarding in most of the classes. This is an essential part of the class. You might find this practice difficult, but we will work on ways to help you manage feelings of distress that come up.

4. **Bringing clutter from home to class**:   In order for you to complete various class assignments we will ask you to bring in a small bag or box of your belongings from home **to every class** starting in the third session. We will use these belongings to demonstrate the skills that you are learning in class. It might be tempting to pre-sort your belongings before class, leaving the "good stuff" at home and only bringing in things that would be easy to discard. For the sake of this practice, we don't want you to pre-sort what you bring in. Just take a handful of belongings from one area of your home, regardless of your thoughts about keeping or discarding them.

5. **Staying on schedule**:   You will notice that your class leaders have a large clock sign. They will use this to help keep class members on track. We have found from our past classes that many class members have important stories to tell, but there often just isn't enough time to get through all of them.

We want to make sure that we stay on track and get through all of the materials that we need to for the class. We will use the clock sign as a reminder for you to finish up with what you are saying quickly (within 30 seconds) and as a signal that we will be moving on.

6. **Progress photos**: An important part of the class is to bring photos from home to demonstrate your homework (discarding). This aspect of the class might also be difficult for you. You might feel embarrassed showing pictures of your home, or you might worry that your pictures won't show enough progress over time. We understand that it can be hard, but in our opinion, taking and showing pictures is very important. It helps to break the wall of secrecy and shame that so often surrounds hoarding, and helps you and us get a good understanding of how well the program is working for you.

CLASS TASK: Introduce Yourself!

Let's start with introductions. Please tell us briefly:

- *Your first name.*
- *Why it is important for you to reduce your clutter right now.*

You can list the class leaders' names and contact information here:

1. _____
Phone:
Email (optional):

_____

2. _____
Phone:
Email (optional):

_____

2.   Class Rules and Guidelines

We find that the Declutter Class works best when we have strict rules and guidelines that everyone in the class follows. On the next few pages you will find a treatment contract and a confidentiality contract. Please read through these contracts and sign the bottom of the form *if you agree to the conditions listed*.

We take the treatment contract and class confidentiality seriously. Unfortunately, if you do not agree to the treatment contract, we are unable to have you in our class. We will take a copy of the signed contract so that we know that you agree to the rules.

The class leaders also have some rules that they will follow:

- *Will not touch any of your possessions without your permission.*
- *Will not throw away any of your possessions without your permission.*
- *Will allow you to make all the decisions about your discarding.*
- *Will be creative and flexible in the treatment process.*
- *Will allow everyone the chance to speak and learn in the class.*
- *Will convey nonjudgmental empathy and compassion, and will strive to understand your situation as accurately as possible.*

Treatment Contract

I _____ *(name) agree to*
the following conditions of the Declutter Class:

1. **Willingness to discard.**   The purpose of this class is to help me to reduce my clutter and improve my quality of life. For this reason, I am willing to discard items in my home. I will be able to control what I keep and discard, but I am open to discarding at least some of the items in my home.

2. **Being on time.**   I understand that if I am 15 minutes or more late to the class (according to the clock in the classroom) I will not be able to attend class that week. If I am less than 15 minutes late the class will not stop to review what I have missed but I may join the class for that week.

3. **Bringing in clutter from home.**   I agree to bring in some of the clutter from my home *to every class* (starting in week 3). This will help me apply and practice the skills from class. This is an extremely important part of the class. I understand that if I do not bring items each week I may be withdrawn from the class.

4. **Maintaining regular attendance.**   I understand that if I miss 3 sessions or am late by 15 minutes or more for 3 sessions I may be asked to leave the class. This is because it is distracting for other class members. If I do miss a class, I understand that I am responsible for contacting the class leaders to find out the homework assignment. Homework must still be completed for missed classes.

5. **Completing assigned home exercises each week.**   I agree to turn in all assigned homework worksheets at each class. If I miss this goal, I understand that I will be asked to meet privately with the class leaders to problem solve any difficulties. If I miss this goal more than 3 times I may be withdrawn from the class.

6. **Focusing on making changes to my current life and not dwelling on past events.**   During the class, I will only bring up past events if it is for the purpose of making changes to my current situation.

7. **Letting others have their turn to speak.**   I will not interrupt others or divert a topic of discussion. I understand that the class leaders will use the clock sign to signal me to finish up what I am saying quickly before moving on to the next topic.

8. **Ceasing all social conversation with other class members by the start of the class.**

9. **Refraining from giving belongings to other class members or acquiring materials from other class members unless instructed by the class leaders as part of demonstration of skills.**

I understand that these rules are for the purpose of helping me with problems associated with hoarding disorder. They are designed to reduce problems that can interfere with my treatment progress. I agree to the above conditions.

Signature: _____   **Date:** _____

Class Confidentiality Contract

This is a contract for confidentiality among the members of this class.

1. Each member of the class agrees to keep personal information discussed in the class private.
2. Any information shared by a class member about himself or herself should be considered private information. This information should not be shared with anyone outside of the class.
3. Due to potential conflicts, we do not recommend contact between class members outside of the class.

   - I agree to respect the right of others to follow this recommendation.
   - I agree to not share contact information while at the class.

Name: _____

Signature: _____

Date: _____

3. What is Hoarding Disorder?

People can be diagnosed with hoarding disorder when they:

1. *Have difficulty discarding possessions.*
2. *Experience distress when trying to discard possessions.*
3. *Have so much clutter that they have trouble using rooms and objects in their home.*

Many people with hoarding disorder also often have a problem of *excessive acquiring*. That is, they buy or pick up more items than they need, and bring them into the home, adding to the clutter. Excessive acquiring isn't one of the diagnostic criteria for hoarding disorder, but we have found it to be present in most cases.

Many people with hoarding disorder report that the saving, acquiring, and clutter in their home can lead to many problems, including:

- Unsanitary and unsafe living conditions
- Difficulties getting contractors or emergency workers into the home
- Arguments with family members
- Reduced social contact
- Financial problems
- Eviction
- Problems with the health department, housing department, fire department, or other agencies
- Dissatisfaction with the functioning of the home
- Losing/being unable to find important items

Frequently Asked Questions About Hoarding Disorder

How common is hoarding disorder?   Hoarding is a common problem around the world. Recent studies suggest that between 2 and 5% of the population experience clinical levels of clutter and could be diagnosed with hoarding disorder.

What is the difference between hoarding disorder and just being messy?   A lot of people have problems with clutter, but not all of these people have hoarding disorder. Hoarding disorder is primarily characterized by difficulty discarding because of a perceived need to save things, or severe emotional distress when discarding. A person could be messy, but if the person doesn't experience difficulty discarding things, we wouldn't describe it as hoarding disorder.

Hoarding disorder is also different from "messiness" in terms of the severity of the clutter. A lot of people have clutter in their homes, and they might find their clutter to be annoying or embarrassing, but hoarding disorder takes it a step further. When someone has hoarding disorder, the clutter is so severe that it gets in the way of them being able to live their life the way they want to.

What do we know about the biological reasons for hoarding?   Research shows that hoarding may partially have a genetic basis. People who have hoarding disorder are more likely to have parents, siblings, or children who also have too much clutter. Brain scans of people with hoarding disorder show that when they have to make decisions about whether to keep or discard possessions, their brains function differently than do the brains of people who do not have hoarding problems. In particular, when people with hoarding disorder have to make decisions about whether to keep or discard their possessions (as you will be doing in this class), their brain reacts as if very serious situation, with great potential for negative consequences. Their brain signals that *everything* is very important, and that makes it harder to let go of things. In this class, we'll help you work through those signals from your brain that tell you to keep things.

What do we know about the psychological reasons for hoarding?   Throughout this class, we'll be talking a lot about the psychological reasons for hoarding. You'll find that understanding and overcoming them is the key to getting the problem under control. In brief, we think that hoarding stems from a combination of problems with:

1. *Decision-making and problem solving:*   It's very common for people with hoarding disorder to have difficulty sustaining attention and making decisions. These issues can make it hard for them to solve problems, make a good plan, and stick to it. You'll see that much of this class is dedicated to helping you make decisions in a more effective and efficient way.

2. *Intense emotions:*   Many people with hoarding disorder find that they struggle with feelings of sadness, anxiety, grief, or anger. These feelings can make it harder for them to make decisions or to let go of their possessions. In this class, we'll show you ways to manage unhappy emotions so they don't control you.

3. *Unhelpful thinking:*   People with hoarding disorder often have strong beliefs about their possessions, some of which might be inaccurate, exaggerated, or just plain unhelpful. Many also feel a strong sense of attachment to objects. In this class, we'll examine your beliefs about possessions and discarding, and will help you think things through more accurately.

4. *Motivation:*   Many people with hoarding problems are ambivalent about cleaning up the clutter. They may think that the problem is not so bad, or that the costs of cleaning up outweigh the potential benefits. Even if your motivation is very high right now, it's quite likely that at some point you'll find your motivation slipping. Throughout the class, we'll use various strategies to help keep your motivation high and encourage you to keep working.

4.   What Will I Learn in This Class?

In this class we will help you to:

1. *Learn more about what contributes to you having clutter.*
2. *Learn evidence-based skills to reduce the clutter in your home.*
3. *Learn how to apply the skills on a consistent basis.*

Learn More About What Contributes to You Having Clutter

As we talked about above, we know that people with hoarding disorder tend to have problems in one or more of the following areas:

1. Decision-making and problem solving
2. Intense emotions
3. Unhelpful thinking
4. Motivation

Difficulties in these four areas lead to acquiring and reluctance to discard. Because everyone is different, we will help you to understand the areas that are problematic for you and to understand the reasons for your own hoarding behavior. We will start to learn more about this in the next class.

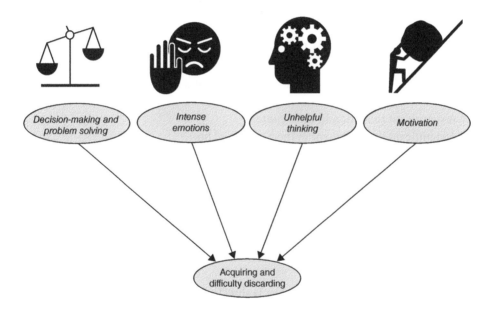

Learn Evidence-Based Skills to Reduce the Clutter in Your Home

The Declutter Class teaches you evidence-based skills to reduce the clutter in your home. We call the skills that we will teach you "evidence-based" because we know from a lot of research that they work! The skills are not easy to do, though, and require lots of repetition and practice. Just like learning any new skill, it also takes time!

We will give you time to practice the skills in class, but it is also important that you practice the skills at home. We recommend spending at least 1 hour a day working on the skills. The more time you spend practicing the skills, the better off you will be at the end of the class.

Sometimes people find some skills work more for them than others. This is normal, but we ask you to at least try all the skills before you decide that they will not work for you. We are confident, however, that if you work on these skills a little bit each day, you will make improvements in your symptoms.

Learn How to Apply the Skills on a Consistent Basis

This is the most important part of the class. From week 11 onwards we will be putting all the skills together and making them part of your everyday life. This takes lots of practice and repetition. After lots of practice with these skills we expect that you will make much improvement in reducing the clutter in your home. You will most likely notice that it is much easier to make decisions about discarding and it will not be as distressing for you to throw items away.

5.   How Well Does the Declutter Class Work?

Past research shows that people who complete a course like this will have:

- A significant reduction in their clutter
- A significant improvement in their quality of life
- Improved safety in their home
- Less buying and acquiring
- Improved ability to organize possessions and to let go of them when necessary

It's important to recognize that simply attending the class will not help the clutter problem. This class will only work if you invest the time and energy needed to do the work outside of class. Research shows us that:

- The amount of benefit you receive is directly related to how much homework you do.
- People who do the best are those who practice the skills regularly.
- Those who continue to practice the skills after the class is finished will continue to reduce the clutter in their homes.

6.   Homework

Doing homework is not always pleasant. It's time consuming and can be difficult, both emotionally and physically. We understand that your life may already be quite busy, and that you may not want to do things that make you feel bad. But we cannot emphasize enough how critical this part of the class is.

We have found from our previous classes that people who do their homework every week get the best outcomes. For example, one recent research study found that 80% of those who did their homework regularly saw a significant benefit from this class. In contrast, only 20% of those who did not do their homework regularly saw a significant benefit. In other words: If you do your homework consistently, you will probably have a very good outcome of this class. If you do *not* do your homework consistently, you will probably *not* have a very good outcome of this class.

For this reason, you will have homework every session. We want you to get the most out of the class so we want you to do your homework every day. If you do not do all your homework consistently, you may be removed from the class (see the class contract). We recommend spending at least 1 hour a day working through your homework.

Your homework this week is:

1. **Reread information from week 1 (including Rita's story).**
2. **Take "before" photos of ALL main areas of your home.**
3. **Complete the "What Has Hoarding Taken From Me?" worksheet.**
4. **Other:** _____
5. **Other:** _____

Rita's Story

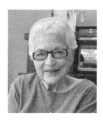

I want to welcome you all to the Declutter Class. I completed the class many months ago now and wanted to let you all know about my experience.

I had a real problem with clutter before I started the class. I would collect way too many things like craft items, knick-knacks, clothes, and books. Over the years things just got out of control. It got to the point where I was unable to use many rooms of my house because it was full of all my stuff.

My family got really annoyed by my stuff (they called it junk). But I had a lot of trouble sorting through things and throwing them away. They offered to help me get rid of things many times but it made me feel like a child and I just got angry at them. It got so bad that my family refused to come around my house any more because they thought it was not safe. That really hurt!

My daughter told me about the Declutter Class. I didn't think that any class could help me reduce my clutter. I felt like I was a lost cause. Initially I just enrolled in the Declutter Class to get her off my back. To my surprise, though, the skills taught in the Declutter Class really helped me to make changes in my life. I was able to gradually work on throwing things away and also bringing less stuff into my home. It's not a miracle cure, though. It was hard work and at times I thought I wouldn't make it through the class and felt like dropping out. But I kept at it and now I can really see the difference. My family can see the difference as well and they are no longer afraid to come to my home.

You will hear from me over the coming weeks. I hope you can learn from me, as well as your class leaders. You might also be able to learn from some of the mistakes I made along the way.

Good luck!
Rita.

What Has Hoarding Taken From Me?

In this class we want you to fight back against what hoarding and clutter has taken from you. An important first step in this process is to identify what the clutter has cost you. Find below some common costs of hoarding. Check the ones that are relevant for you.

Family
- ☐ Family can no longer come to your home
- ☐ Arguments with family members
- ☐ Less time with family
- ☐ Loss of custody of a child or elder
- ☐ Other _____

Social
- ☐ Friends can no longer come to your home
- ☐ You have let friendships go because of the state of your home
- ☐ Arguments with friends because of the state of your home
- ☐ Less time with friends
- ☐ Disagreements or strained relationships with neighbors
- ☐ Other _____

Health
- ☐ Problems breathing
- ☐ Bed bugs or other bugs
- ☐ Skin problems
- ☐ Rodents in the home
- ☐ Emergency services unable to come in and help in an emergency
- ☐ Unable to get out of the home quickly in a fire
- ☐ Other _____

Emotional
- ☐ Anger
- ☐ Sadness
- ☐ Anxiety
- ☐ Frustration
- ☐ Other _____

Economic/legal
- ☐ Spent more money than you can afford
- ☐ Borrowed money from others that you can't pay back
- ☐ Debt problems
- ☐ Trouble with state/government agencies due to clutter
- ☐ Evicted or threatened with eviction
- ☐ Other _____

Valuing your time and money

- ☐ Over the past year, how many hours do you think you have wasted acquiring items, looking for lost items, or being otherwise inconvenienced by clutter? _____

- ☐ How much do you think an hour of your time is worth? That is, if someone wanted to buy one hour of your life, what would you charge for it? $_____

- ☐ How much has hoarding cost you in terms of personal time over the past year? $_____

- ☐ How much money have you spent rebuying items that you already had, or buying things you did not use? $_____

Other

- ☐ _____
- ☐ _____
- ☐ _____

Why Do I Have So Much Stuff?

1.   Homework Review

As we mentioned in the last class, homework is a very important part of the class. Research shows that people in the class who do regular homework do much better than people who don't. This is why we regularly monitor your homework and why

CBT for Hoarding Disorder: A Group Therapy Program Workbook, First Edition. David F. Tolin, Bethany M. Wootton, Blaise L. Worden, and Christina M. Gilliam.
© 2017 John Wiley & Sons Ltd. Published 2017 by John Wiley & Sons Ltd.

we provide rewards when you do your homework (you'll find out more about this later in this class).

In order to monitor your homework, we will spend time at the start of each class talking about your homework and we will decide as a class **whether your homework goals have been met**.

CLASS TASK: Homework Review

Everyone take out their **homework sheets** from last week. We will go around the class and discuss whether each person completed their homework tasks. The homework tasks from last week are listed below. Please indicate which of these tasks you completed over the past week.

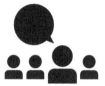

1. **Reread information from week 1 (including Rita's story).**
2. **Take "before" photos of ALL main areas of your home.**
3. **Complete the "What Has Hoarding Taken From Me?" worksheet.**
4. **Other:** _____
5. **Other:** _____

Now let's talk about rewards.

2.   Rewards

We believe that rewards are an important part of helping people to maintain motivation. We also know from lots of research that whenever someone has a personal goal – whether it's to quit smoking, to lose weight, or to declutter their home – they are much more likely to stick with the program when they can give themselves small rewards along the way. That's true for kids, adults, even your class leaders. We all need encouragement when we're doing something that's hard. In this class we use both individual and class rewards to help keep your motivation high.

Individual Rewards

Each week as part of the homework review we will discuss as a class whether you met your homework goals (we call these SMART goals and you will learn more about them today). For us to review how you are doing you must show us your progress by regularly taking photos of the area of your home that you are working on (before and after photos).

When you complete your SMART goal, we want you to reward yourself – not by buying or otherwise acquiring more stuff, but rather with a pleasant activity that you don't normally do. This may be something like:

- Going to a movie
- Going on a day trip somewhere special
- Having a nice dinner
- Watching your favorite TV show
- Visiting a friend

So let's talk about some ways that you can reward yourself for meeting your goals.

CLASS TASK: Brainstorm Rewards

As a class let's come up with some pleasant things that you might like to do as your reward for meeting your SMART goal. They can include things that don't cost any money. If a class member mentions something that you think would interest you, write it in the space below.

1. _____   2. _____

3. _____   4. _____

5. _____   6. _____

7. _____   8. _____

9. _____   10. _____

Class Rewards

In addition to the individual rewards, by achieving their SMART goal each class member will also contribute to a class reward. In order for the class to get a reward point, 75% of the class need to have completed their SMART goal. The class leaders will keep track of the class's progress.

When 6 points have been earned, each class member will be provided with:

_____

Once the first reward is received the reward will then reset and you will work toward a second reward. You will need another 6 points to reach this reward. The second reward will be:

_____

We have found from our past classes that most class members enjoy these rewards, and that working as a class toward rewards helps to keep motivation high.

Now let's learn more about why clutter is a problem for you.

3.   Meet the Bad Guys

We know from past research that people with hoarding disorder tend to have problems in one or more of the following areas:

1.   *Decision-making and problem solving*
2.   *Intense emotions*
3.   *Unhelpful thinking*
4.   *Waxing and waning motivation*

Difficulties in these four areas lead to acquiring and difficulty discarding.

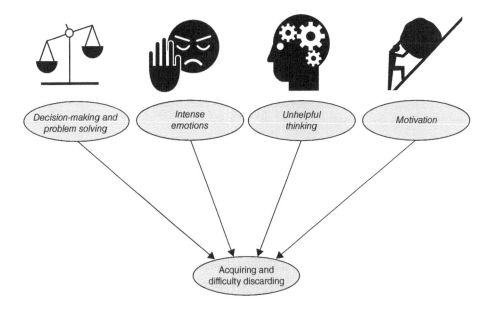

Decision-Making and Problem Solving

There is a lot of research to show that people with hoarding disorder tend to have problems with skills like decision-making and problem solving. For example, in terms of acquiring, people often:

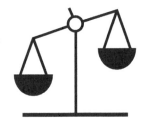

• Leave the house without a plan about what to buy (which results in buying other unneeded items).

- Focus on the positive aspects of the object without considering other relevant factors (e.g., focusing on the sale price of an item and ignoring that they don't need the item at all).
- Buy something that they already have but can't find because of the clutter.

And in terms of discarding, people often:

- Have difficulties making decisions about what item to start with when trying to discard.
- Tell stories about the item rather than making decisions about where the item belongs.
- Get distracted by other things rather than focusing on the item in their hand.
- Become involved in other people's belongings instead of their own.
- Jump from one section of their home to another, never making any progress in one area of discarding.
- Move items from pile to pile without actually removing them from the home (we call this "churning").
- Spend excessive amounts of time making decisions about possessions.

An important part of the class is to teach you how to improve your decision-making and problem-solving skills in order to reduce the clutter in your home.

Intense Emotions

Emotions are a normal part of life and everyone feels various emotions throughout the day. However, emotions can become problematic when we let them influence our behavior in a way that is not helpful to us.

Individuals with hoarding disorder tend to collect belongings because it makes some kind of emotional distress less severe. For example, they might go and buy things to make a bad feeling (such as guilt or sadness) go away. They may also avoid discarding in order to avoid the negative feelings that go along with discarding.

Some common intense emotions in people with hoarding disorder include:

- **Anxiety**
- **Sadness**
- **Anger**
- **Loneliness**
- **Grief**
- **Guilt**

A big part of this class is learning skills to help you to identify your emotion better, and to cope with these intense emotions in more adaptive ways.

Unhelpful Thinking

We have known for a long time that the way we think about things determines how we feel about them. For example, imagine that a family member offered to help you with clearing your house.

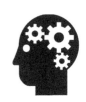

If you thought...	You would probably feel...
"She's always judging me"	Angry
"Maybe she won't come around any more if I don't clean up the house"	Anxious
"I'll never be able to get through all this stuff"	Sad
"What a great help that would be. I could get through things much faster with some help"	Happy

So even in the same situation a person can have different thoughts, which leads to different emotional responses. There are many ways to think about a particular situation, and our way of thinking about it might not be "the truth." We can step back and investigate our thoughts about discarding and acquiring to see if they are accurate or if they are leading us astray and making us feel worse.

An important part of this class is learning skills to help you reduce the unhelpful thoughts and help you use more adaptive ways of thinking to improve your discarding and reduce your acquiring.

Waxing and Waning Motivation

Research shows us that people with hoarding disorder tend to have trouble maintaining motivation to sort and make decisions about their belongings. Often we see that motivation goes up and down over the 16 weeks of the class.

Most often, people are highly motivated at the start of the class. Later on, when you might notice your motivation slipping, we'll include some exercises to help keep you going.

Another important part of this class is to help you to improve and maintain your motivation to reduce your clutter.

Everyone is different and the extent to which these issues (or bad guys) are important for each class member will vary. It is important to identify which of the above issues is a problem for you. This way you will know what to focus most on in the treatment.

Over the next few weeks you will develop skills to address each of the bad guys. We will cover the following topics over the remaining class lessons:

Week 3	Making Decisions and Solving Problems: Part 1
Week 4	Making Decisions and Solving Problems: Part 2
Week 5	Intense Emotions: Part 1
Week 6	Intense Emotions: Part 2
Week 7	Unhelpful Thinking: Part 1
Week 8	Unhelpful Thinking: Part 2
Week 9	Waxing and Waning Motivation: Part 1
Week 10	Waxing and Waning Motivation: Part 2
Week 11	Putting It All Together: Part 1
Week 12	Putting It All Together: Part 2
Week 13	Putting It All Together: Part 3
Week 14	Putting It All Together: Part 4
Week 15	Staying Clutter Free in the Future: Part 1
Week 16	Staying Clutter Free in the Future: Part 2

CLASS TASK: Identifying Your Bad Guys

In this class task we would like you to start to understand how much each of the bad guys impacts your own hoarding behavior. Rate how much you think each of the bad guys is impacting your acquiring and difficulty discarding below.

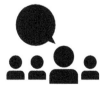

Decision-making and problem solving

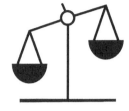

Acquiring: *How much do you think problems with decision-making and problem solving are getting in the way and are affecting your acquiring? How much do you notice that you are unable to weigh up the pros and cons and think through your decision when you want to acquire an item?*

0 —— 1 —— 2 —— 3 —— 4 —— 5 —— 6 —— 7 —— 8 —— 9 —— 10

0 = Not a problem for me
10 = A very big problem for me

Discarding: *How much do you think that problems with making decisions and problem solving are getting in the way of your discarding? How much do you notice that you want to sift through your belongings rather than focus on one particular item and make a decision about it? How much do you notice your mind wandering, rather than making a decision about the item? Are you changing your mind back and forth about whether or not you should keep the object?*

0 —— 1 —— 2 —— 3 —— 4 —— 5 —— 6 —— 7 —— 8 —— 9 —— 10

0 = Not a problem for me
10 = A very big problem for me

Intense emotions

Acquiring: *What kinds of emotions are you feeling when you acquire something? Interested? Excited? What kinds of emotions do you think you will experience if you don't obtain this object? Guilty? Sad? Bored? How much are these intense emotions contributing to your acquiring behavior?*

0 —— 1 —— 2 —— 3 —— 4 —— 5 —— 6 —— 7 —— 8 —— 9 —— 10

0 = Not a problem for me
10 = A very big problem for me

Discarding: *What kinds of emotions are you feeling when you are discarding? What emotions do you think you will feel after you discard an object? Sadness? Grief? Anger? Frustration? Anxiety? Guilt? How much are these emotions getting in the way of you being able to discard as much as you would like to?*

0 —— 1 —— 2 —— 3 —— 4 —— 5 —— 6 —— 7 —— 8 —— 9 —— 10

0 = Not a problem for me
10 = A very big problem for me

Unhelpful thinking

Acquiring: When you are faced with a situation where you want to acquire, what is going through your mind? How much are you experiencing unhelpful thoughts? Are you thinking that you might have a good use for the item? Are you thinking that you shouldn't pass up such a great deal?

0 —— 1 —— 2 —— 3 —— 4 —— 5 —— 6 —— 7 —— 8 —— 9 —— 10

0 = Not a problem for me
10 = A very big problem for me

Discarding: When you are discarding, what is going through your mind? How much are you experiencing unhelpful thoughts? Are you thinking the item will be useful? Or that you're being wasteful? Or that you could give the item to a friend?

0 —— 1 —— 2 —— 3 —— 4 —— 5 —— 6 —— 7 —— 8 —— 9 —— 10

0 = Not a problem for me
10 = A very big problem for me

Waxing and waning motivation

Acquiring: How much do you think low motivation is getting in the way of you resisting acquiring? In other words, are you feeling like you don't want to work on your clutter problem right now?

0 —— 1 —— 2 —— 3 —— 4 —— 5 —— 6 —— 7 —— 8 —— 9 —— 10

0 = Not a problem for me
10 = A very big problem for me

Discarding: How much do you think low motivation is getting in the way of you discarding? In other words, are you feeling unmotivated to work on your discarding right now? Or are you thinking that maybe your clutter isn't such a big problem after all?

0 —— 1 —— 2 —— 3 —— 4 —— 5 —— 6 —— 7 —— 8 —— 9 —— 10

0 = Not a problem for me
10 = A very big problem for me

4.   Setting Goals

Setting goals and working toward them is an important part of reducing your clutter. Part of what we will do today is to teach you how to set long-term goals (what you would like to achieve by the end of the class) as well as short-term goals (such as a weekly homework goal). Each week you will work toward a short-term goal related to discarding, which should be aimed at reducing the clutter in your home. Meeting the short-term goals will help you to achieve your long-term goals and will also help you to obtain your individual and class rewards.

SMART Goals

When you set goals it's best that they are SMART goals:

S   *Specific*
M   *Measurable*
A   *Attainable*
R   *Relevant*
T   *Time limited*

For example, a goal of "Get the entire house uncluttered and spotless by next week" is not attainable. A goal of "Get the house uncluttered enough to make me happy" is not specific. A goal of "Help my sister mow the lawn" is not relevant to your discarding.

Here are some examples of good long-term SMART goals that relate to discarding:

- Declutter all my kitchen cabinets by the end of the class.
- Have my dining room clear for Thanksgiving.
- Clear enough space for the plumber to be able to enter my home and fix the kitchen sink within 3 months.

Here are some examples of good short-term SMART goals that relate to discarding:

- Discard five inches of paperwork this week.
- Take two bags of clothing to a charity every week.
- Throw away five magazines each day.

A helpful tip to keep in mind is that you should be at least 80% sure that you can reach your goal. If you set your goal too high, you will lose motivation because you will be unlikely to achieve it. If you set your goal too low, you will feel like you are not getting anywhere.

CLASS TASK: Setting SMART Goals

An important first step in decreasing your clutter is to set some goals.

Take a moment now to think about your long-term SMART goals. What do you want to achieve in the course of this group? Write down some long-term goals below.

1. _____

2. _____

3. _____

Each week you will be asked to set a short-term SMART goal as part of your homework. These goals should follow the SMART formula and should involve some quantity of discarding. These SMART goals can work toward the longer-term goals you wrote above.

Let's practice setting these goals now and making sure that they follow the SMART formula. Take a moment to think about your goal for the week. Then we will review these goals. You can write your goal down on the next page in the box – you will have a page like this to write down your goal each week.

5. Homework

Remember that people who do the most homework do the best at the end of the class. We recommend spending at least 1 hour a day working through all your homework tasks (at least 30 minutes of this should be working specifically on your discarding).

This week you will start using the In and Out Log. This is located at the end of this chapter and is something that you will use throughout the remaining weeks of the class. We want you to write down all the things that you bring into the home and all the things that you discard from the home. This will help us to monitor your progress and make sure that you are on track.

Your homework this week is:

1. **Reread information from week 2 (including Rita's story).**
2. **Practice using the In and Out Log every day.**
3. **Practice discarding for a minimum of 30 minutes per day.**
4. **Complete weekly SMART goal.**
5. **Bring items from home to class next week.**
6. **Other:** _____

My SMART goal for this week:
_____

What will be my personal reward for completing my SMART goal this week?
Reward: _____

When will I give myself the reward?
Day: _____

Did I accomplish my SMART goal?   Yes   No
If no, what got in the way? _____

Rita's Story

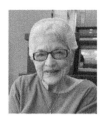

Hi everyone. I found that learning about the bad guys was really useful, but it took me a while to get it. Once I could identify the bad guys I paid close attention to them when I attempted to throw things away at home outside of class.

I noticed that I had a lot of problems with unhelpful thoughts, like thinking that I needed to keep the objects because they reminded me of important times in my life, or thinking that I needed to keep things because I might be able to use them someday.

I also noticed that I had trouble making decisions when I was trying to discard; my mind kept wandering to other topics such as all of the other things I needed to do that day, and even when I was focusing on the item in front of me, I was at a loss for where to put it or how to decide whether it was really important to me.

I could also relate to the intense emotions information: When I was considering throwing something away, I felt very sad and guilty, like I was doing something wrong or bad. The thought of throwing away something that I might need also made me quite anxious because I don't like to be unprepared – I'm just not that kind of person.

I felt like my motivation was good when I first started the class, although I did notice at times it wasn't always as good as it could be. When I noticed that my motivation was lacking I went back and had a look at the worksheet from the first class – the one on what the clutter has cost me – and I also reminded myself of my long-term SMART goals.

My first short-term SMART goal was to clear a small section of my kitchen counter (the size of a dinner plate) within a week. That was much easier than trying to handle the whole house! I felt good when I achieved it and I enjoyed my reward (which was a nice coffee and cake at my local café).

Good luck. I hope that you can achieve your goals this week!
Rita.

In and Out Log – Week 2 Example

Date	In	Out
Monday	• Coffee cup • Cat food • mouthwash (2) • oatmeal • 5 pieces of mail • Birthday cards (2) • Shampoo and conditioner • Body lotion (10) • Chapstick • Cat litter • Hand soap refill	• 10 articles of clothes to charity • Old car maintenance records • Box of sweets • Expired cans of food (5)

In and Out Log – Week 2

Date	In	Out

Chapter 3/16

Making Decisions
and Solving Problems

Part 1

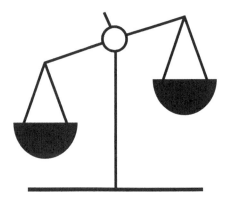

Overview

CBT for Hoarding Disorder: A Group Therapy Program Workbook, First Edition. David F. Tolin,
Bethany M. Wootton, Blaise L. Worden, and Christina M. Gilliam.
© 2017 John Wiley & Sons Ltd. Published 2017 by John Wiley & Sons Ltd.

1. Homework Review

CLASS TASK: Homework Review

We will go around the class and discuss each class member's homework and whether they have achieved their personal reward and contributed to the class reward for this week.

The homework tasks from last week were:

1. **Reread information from week 2 (including Rita's story).**
2. **Practice using the In and Out Log every day.**
3. **Practice discarding for a minimum of 30 minutes per day.**
4. **Complete weekly SMART goal.**
5. **Bring items from home to class next week.**
6. **Other:** _____

- Did you accomplish your SMART goal for the week? If not, how will you change things to make it more likely you will succeed this week? **Remember that the more you practice the skills, the better you will be at the end of the class!**
- Did you reward yourself? **Remember that rewards help to keep your motivation high.**

_____
_____
_____
_____
_____

2. Making Decisions and Solving Problems

There are a number of ways that problems with decision-making and problem solving can lead to difficulty with discarding. We will talk about a few of them in this class. You may find that some relate to you more than others. We will also discuss this further in the next class. Some of the things that can get in the way when trying to discard include the following:

- Not knowing how much stuff is too much stuff to keep.
- Not being able to find the time to discard.
- Not knowing where things go.
- Not having a system for discarding.
- Not knowing how to solve problems that come up when discarding.

In this class and the next one we will learn skills to address each of these obstacles. We know that not all of these issues will apply to all people in the class, but we ask you to give each of these skills a try before focusing on the ones that are most relevant for you.

Obstacle		*Skill that you will learn*
Not knowing how much stuff is too much stuff to keep ...		**Guidelines for Discarding**
Not being able to find the time to discard ...		**Time Scheduling**
Not knowing where things go ...		**Improving Organization**
Not having a system for discarding...		**Discarding Flowchart**
Not knowing how to solve problems that come up when discarding ...		**Problem Solving (week 4)**

Let's start.

3.   Guidelines for Discarding

Often people with hoarding disorder tell us that they are not exactly sure how to go about discarding. For this reason we developed 10 guidelines to help you with sorting and discarding. These guidelines will help you to get the most out of your sorting and discarding sessions.

1. **Take regular photos so that you can see your progress.**   Often people forget what their home first looked like, so they forget or don't see the good work they are doing when discarding. We have already asked you to take a "before" photo of each room in your home. We recommend that you take photos of the same room every few weeks to see all the positive changes that you have made.

2. **OHIO – Only Handle It Once.**   When you are working your way through your belongings it is important that once you have made a decision on something, you stick to it. Also, if you pick something up, you make a decision about it immediately – you can't put it back down and say, "I'll deal with this later." For example, if something goes in the recycling, then it stays in the

recycling. Or if you pick up an important magazine, then you make a decision about the important magazine immediately. Using the OHIO rule (**O**nly **H**andle **I**t **O**nce) will help you get through the greatest amount of your belongings as possible and help you to learn how to make decisions about things more effectively.

3. **Get it out of the house.**   Often when people decide to donate or recycle an item they will forget to take it to the final location (e.g., a charity or the recycling depot). An important rule for effective discarding is to remove these items from your home as soon as possible (set a time limit). It may be helpful to schedule some time through the week to drop off your donation or recycling items and to do it the same day and time each week so that it becomes part of your routine. The nice thing about using boxes, rather than piles, is that the box has a built-in signal. When no more will fit in the box, stop and move the box to where it goes.

4. **Work on the same area.**   When people are working on their sorting and discarding, they often move between different areas of their house – for example, working in the kitchen one day, then the garage the next day, then the patio the day after that. Rather than spending 30 minutes each day on a different area of your house, we recommend that you focus on one area until that area is clear. This will allow you to see the progress that you are making and will help to boost motivation.

5. **Choose a highly visible area.**   When you are choosing the area to work on, it is important that you choose a highly visible area in your home (such as a main room or hallway) rather than choosing an area of your home that you will never see (like inside a closet). Working on these types of areas will help you to see your progress, and again, this will provide you with extra motivation.

6. **Don't churn.**   When you have picked the area that you are going to work on, it is important that you spend the full 30 minutes actually working on sorting and discarding items in your home rather than just picking things up and putting them down on a different pile. We call this "churning." We want you to pick up the first thing you see and make a decision *quickly* about it and then move on to the next item.

7. **Throw it away (especially if it is damaged).**   People with hoarding disorder frequently say that they prefer to donate items than to throw them in the trash. Often donating items makes people feel less intense emotions than throwing them away. However, donating means that you have an extra step when you are discarding (going to goodwill or the second-hand store) and can be an extra hurdle that you don't need. For this reason it is often preferable to throw items in the trash rather than trying to donate them. If your item is damaged in any way – stained, has holes in it, or is not working properly – then it is best just to throw it away rather than trying to give it to

someone else or donate it. Many donation sites also do not accept or will discard nonworking or damaged items, so save yourself the time and effort by just throwing it in the trash.

8. **Be your own cheerleader.**   Often people with hoarding disorder are their own worst critic. As we talked about in the last class, thinking unhelpful thoughts leads to negative emotions and negative emotions can lead to poor motivation. We want you to be your own cheerleader – be as kind to yourself as you would someone else in the same situation. Would you tell someone else in the class that there is no point, so stop trying? No – so don't say it to yourself! Make sure you give yourself the kind of encouragement that you would give to another class member and remember to reward yourself for a successful discarding session.

9. **Schedule discarding sessions.**   It is important that you schedule time into your day to practice sorting and discarding. If you do not schedule this time into your day, you may find that all the other things you need to do in the day get done, but you have not practiced your sorting and discarding. Scheduling the time allows you to make sure everything gets done. We will learn more about scheduling later in this class.

10. **The 12-month rule.**   A lot of people have found it helpful to have a 12-month rule. This means that if you haven't used the item in the past 12 months, then get rid of it.

CLASS TASK: Making Your Own Guidelines

These are the 10 guidelines that we have found to be most helpful for other people with hoarding disorder. Everyone is different, though, and you may have some other guidelines that are relevant for you. Please list these guidelines below and share them with the class – because you may find that other people have the need for the same guideline.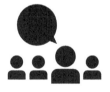

My <u>extra</u> guidelines for sorting and discarding:

_____

_____

_____

_____

_____

4. Scheduling the Time to Work on Discarding

We know from research that people who spend the most time on sorting and discarding are the people who tend to be doing the best at the end of the class. But we also realize that people are busy and may not know when to schedule time in their busy day to work on their discarding. As part of your homework you have been asked to work on discarding for 30 minutes per day (or 3.5 hours a week). Many of you may like to work on discarding for more than that and that's great, but we recommend 30 minutes per day at a *minimum*. You may also find it helpful to set a number of items to discard in each sorting and discarding session. This will make it less likely for you to just churn during sorting and discarding (moving things from one spot to another without discarding anything) and will help you to reach your SMART goal each week.

In order to schedule the best time to discard, we recommend that you:

1. **Find the best time *for you.*** Some people like to work on their discarding first thing in the morning to get it out of the way. However, other people say that they like to do their discarding at another time of the day. We recommend that you think about the things you do regularly through the day (such as watching your favorite night-time show) and agree that you will do that *only* after you have completed your discarding homework.

2. **Pick a time of the day when there are minimal distractions.** It's best to work on your sorting and discarding when you won't be distracted by other people. For example, a time of day when your children or spouse are not home would be preferable. Remember that you have the power to *reduce distractions* by turning off the phone ringer, the television, etc. You also can add things that will help keep you motivated or relaxed, such as your favorite music.

3. **Break down your scheduled discarding sessions to multiple, shorter sessions, if the thought of sorting and discarding for 30 minutes is too overwhelming.** We recommend that you dedicate *at least 30 minutes daily*, at a minimum, to sorting and discarding in order for your treatment to be successful. If this seems impossible, schedule three (or more) 10-minute sessions each day. You also can use this strategy on days when you are feeling overwhelmed or unmotivated to sort/discard for 30 minutes in one sitting. You may want to set a timer for 10 minutes and sort/discard until the timer goes off. Over time, you can gradually increase your sorting/discarding time with this strategy.

4. **Pencil it in.** Use a calendar or daily planner in order to help you schedule the best time for discarding for you. Once you schedule in a time, stick to it. Don't put it off.

An important way to find time to work on discarding is to schedule your day so that you make sure you have factored your discarding around your other commitments. We will talk more about this later, but in order for you to make the most out of the

Scheduling in Discarding Times: Example

	Monday	Tuesday	Wednesday	Thursday	Friday	Saturday	Sunday
5 am–6 am	Sleep	Sleep	Sleep	Sleep	Sleep	Sleep	Sleep
6 am–7 am	Get ready	Get ready	Get ready	Get ready	Get ready	Sleep	Sleep
7 am–8 am	Drive to work	Drive to work	Drive to work	Drive to work	Drive to work	Sleep	Sleep
8 am–9 am	Work	Work	Work	Work	Work	TV/breakfast	TV/breakfast
9 am–10 am	Work	Work	Work	Work	Work	DISCARD	DISCARD
10 am–11 am	Work	Work	Work	Work	Work	Get ready	
11 am–12 pm	Work	Work	Work	Work	Work	Drive	
12 pm–1 pm	Work	Work	Work	Work	Work	Lunch/friends	
1 pm–2 pm	Work	Work	Work	Work	Work	Lunch/friends	
2 pm–3 pm	Work	Work	Work	Work	Work		
3 pm–4 pm	Work	Work	Work	Work	Work		
4 pm–5 pm	To home	To home	To home	To home	To home		

5 pm–6 pm	DISCARD	DISCARD	DISCARD	DISCARD	DISCARD
6 pm–7 pm	Dinner	Dinner	Dinner	Dinner	Dinner
7 pm–8 pm	Relax/TV	Relax/TV	Relax/TV	Relax/TV	Relax/TV
8 pm–9 pm	Ready 4 bed	Ready 4 bed	Ready 4 bed	Ready 4 bed	Ready 4 bed
9 pm–10 pm	Read/TV	Read/TV	Read/TV	Read/TV	Read/TV
10 pm–11 pm	Bed	Bed	Bed	Bed	TV
11 pm–12 am	Sleep	Sleep	Sleep	Sleep	TV
12 am–1 am	Sleep	Sleep	Sleep	Sleep	Sleep
1 am–2 am	Sleep	Sleep	Sleep	Sleep	Sleep
2 am–3 am	Sleep	Sleep	Sleep	Sleep	Sleep

Scheduling in Discarding Times

	Monday	Tuesday	Wednesday	Thursday	Friday	Saturday	Sunday
5 am–6 am							
6 am–7 am							
7 am–8 am							
8 am–9 am							
9 am–10 am							
10 am–11 am							
11 am–12 pm							
12 pm–1 pm							
1 pm–2 pm							
2 pm–3 pm							
3 pm–4 pm							

4 pm–5 pm						
5 pm–6 pm						
6 pm–7 pm						
7 pm–8 pm						
8 pm–9 pm						
9 pm–10 pm						
10 pm–11 pm						
11 pm–12 am						
12 am–1 am						
1 am–2 am						
2 am–3 am						

class, sorting and discarding need to be your main priority. As we have talked about before, using small rewards can give you an important boost in motivation.

CLASS TASK: Identifying the Best Time for Discarding and Planning Your Day

Make a plan around when is the best time to practice.

1. What is the time of the day when you are most motivated?

    _____

2. What time of the day do you have least distractions?

    _____

3. What works for you? One 30-minute block or three 10-minute sessions?

    _____

Use this information to schedule sorting and discarding sessions in your daily planner (next page). Use the daily planner to schedule your day for tomorrow so that you are able to fit in all your commitments, including your sorting and discarding. Then each day schedule sorting and discarding for the next day, and so on.

Improving Organization

To help you learn how to improve organization, we will introduce two skills today:

*   How much is too much?
*   Where do things belong?

Let's start.

How Much is Too Much?

People in our past classes have often indicated that they are not sure how much is too much to keep of certain items. For instance, how many old newspapers should someone keep? How many years of receipts should someone hold on to? How many sweaters should someone own? How many tote bags should someone have? How many couches should someone have in their house? While understanding how much is too much is based on many factors (such as how much space and money someone has), coming up with some general rules can also be helpful.

Spend some time as a class discussing how much is too much of different items.

CLASS TASK: Identifying if I Have Too Much Stuff

The first thing to do is to list the things that you often have too much of in your home. Be specific here (i.e., instead of "furniture" indicate the type of furniture ("sofa," "bed," "chairs," etc.).

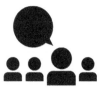

Then as a class decide how much is too much of that item. You will see an example below of someone talking about how many newspapers is too many.

Example:

Items	How much is reasonable?
Newspaper	3 papers

Item:

1.	
2.	
3.	
4.	
5.	
6.	
7.	
8.	
9.	
10.	

Where Do Things Belong?

Often when things have been in the wrong place for a long time people forget where things actually go. It is important that all items in your home have a place so that you can find them and know where to put them when you have made more progress with clearing your home. Some common categories and locations for possessions are outlined below.

Categories	*Where it belongs*
Mail and miscellaneous paper	File cabinets, drawers in office
Magazines	Shelves
Photos	Drawers, boxes, photo albums
Newspapers	Recycle box
Clothing	Drawers in bedroom, closets, laundry basket
Coats	Closets, clothes rack in bedroom
Boots and shoes	Closets, shoe rack in bedroom
Books	Bookshelves
Audio and videotapes	Shelves, drawers
Souvenirs and knick-knacks	Display cabinets, drawers
Decorative items	On display
Office supplies	Desk drawer, shelf, top of desk in office area
Games	Shelves, cabinets
Hardware	Basement, garage, kitchen drawer
Furniture	Placed in appropriate room
Empty containers	Cupboards, basement, garage
Food	Refrigerator, cupboard, pantry
Kitchen utensils	Drawers, containers in kitchen
Pots, pans, and dishes	Cupboards, on hooks in kitchen
Linens	Dining room/bathroom cabinet, linen closet
Toiletries	Bathroom shelves, cabinets or drawers
Cleaning products	Kitchen, bath or laundry cabinet
Cleaning tools (e.g., broom, mop)	Closet, garage or basement
Garden and yard tools	Garage, basement
Recreation equipment	Garage, basement, attic, closet
Paint and equipment	Garage, basement
Pet food and equipment	Closet, cupboard
Handicrafts	Cabinet, shelf, basement

CLASS TASK: Make Your Own Categories

If you have a lot of belongings that don't fall into these categories then you will need to come up with some of your own. Discuss as a class the stuff that you have and where in your home it belongs.

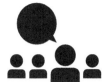

Categories	Where it belongs

5. Putting Skills Together to Discard Better

Follow the Flowchart for Discarding

It can also be useful to follow a flowchart to help you see what you need to do with your belongings. This flowchart provides the basics on *how* to discard. Over the coming weeks you will learn more skills to help you discard.

Step 1: Select an item from your belongings to work on.
Step 2: Make a decision about whether to discard the item or not.

- If you choose to discard the item, you need to figure out which box it belongs in (trash, recycle, or donation). Well done for making this decision.
- If you choose to keep the item, you need to figure out where it belongs (use the categories worksheet from this class to help you decide). You then need to move it to the appropriate location in your home. If space is available, place the item where it belongs. If it isn't, then you need to make a choice about whether you keep the item or not.

Use the flowchart to help you make decisions about this.

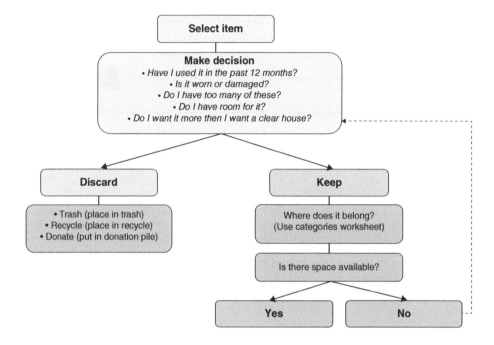

CLASS TASK: Using the Flowchart to Help with Discarding

As a class, spend some time working through the discarding flowchart as you practice sorting through your possessions from home. Discuss any problems that come up with your class leaders.

6.   Homework

Remember that people who do the most homework do the best at the end of the class. We recommend spending at least 1 hour a day working through your homework (at least 30 minutes of this should be spent specifically on discarding).

Your homework this week is:

1.   **Reread information from week 3 (including Rita's story).**
2.   **Practice using the In and Out Log every day.**
3.   **Practice discarding for a minimum of 30 minutes per day (or equivalent).**
4.   **Complete weekly SMART goal.**
5.   **Bring items from home to class next week.**
6.   **Other:** _____

My SMART goal for this week:
_____

What will be my personal reward for completing my SMART goal this week?
Reward: _____

When will I give myself the reward?
Day: _____

Did I accomplish my SMART goal?   Yes   No
If no, what got in the way? _____

Rita's Story

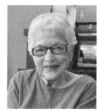

Hi everyone. This week you learned a lot of practical skills to help with discarding. For me, I found it helpful to remember the 10 guidelines, and I used the categories sheet and the discarding flowchart to help me make decisions about where things go, and whether to get rid of things. It wasn't easy, though, and I noticed that some days were tougher than others to discard things.

On the days that were tough I decided to break up my discarding into two 15-minute sessions. This seemed to work well for me. On the days when things were going well, I tried to do more than the minimum 30 minutes.

I realized that a big part of my problem with finding things was that nothing was in its proper "home" – my shoes, for example, were everywhere, which made it hard for me to find them when I needed them. When I put them all in one place they were so much easier to find and use! I also noticed that I probably had way too many pairs of shoes (and probably needed to discard some)!

The skills that you are learning now are very new, so it will take time to learn and master them. Be kind to yourself and be your own cheerleader. Remember to set time to discard and remember to follow the 10 guidelines!

Good luck this week.
Rita.

In and Out Log – Week 3

Date	In	Out

Chapter 4/16

Making Decisions and Solving Problems

Part 2

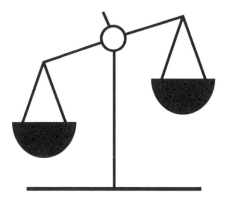

CBT for Hoarding Disorder: A Group Therapy Program Workbook, First Edition. David F. Tolin, Bethany M. Wootton, Blaise L. Worden, and Christina M. Gilliam.
© 2017 John Wiley & Sons Ltd. Published 2017 by John Wiley & Sons Ltd.

1.   Homework Review

CLASS TASK: Homework Review

We will now go around the class and discuss each person's homework and whether they have achieved their SMART goal.

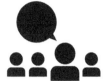

The homework tasks from last week were:

1. **Reread information from week 3 (including Rita's story).**
2. **Practice using the In and Out Log every day.**
3. **Practice discarding for a minimum of 30 minutes per day (or equivalent).**
4. **Complete weekly SMART goal.**
5. **Bring items from home to class next week.**
6. **Other:** _____

- Did you accomplish your SMART goal for the week? If not, how will you change things to make it more likely you will succeed this week? **Remember that the more you practice the skills, the better you will be at the end of the class!**
- Did you reward yourself? **Remember that rewards help to keep your motivation high.**

_____

_____

_____

_____

_____

Now let's learn more about how problems with being focused can cause you to acquire.

2.   Making Decisions: Acquiring

As we discussed last week, many people with hoarding disorder tend to have difficulties with making decisions and solving problems. There are many ways that problems with these skills can contribute to acquiring. In this lesson we will learn some practical skills to help you improve your ability to make decisions, solve problems, and resist acquiring.

The first thing we will learn about is how to recognize high-risk situations for acquiring.

Understanding High-Risk Situations

When people are trying to reduce any unhelpful behavior (such as acquiring or reducing smoking or drinking) one of the most helpful initial steps is to avoid high-risk situations. These can be both internal (an emotional state, like feeling sad) or external (people/places/things).

Some of the more common internal high-risk triggers include emotion states or moods like:

- Feeling lonely
- Feeling sad
- Feeling worried
- Feeling happy
- Feeling bored

Some of the more common external high-risk triggers include the following.

People
- Shopping with a particular person
- Seeing a person who often likes to give you gifts or things to take home
- Family members who also have problems with hoarding disorder

Places
- Dollar stores
- Supermarkets
- Thrift stores/second-hand stores
- Tag sales/garage sales
- Art/craft stores
- Internet shopping
- TV shopping channel/catalogs
- Free items (such as things left curbside)
- Discount/wholesale clubs

Situations
- Sales
- Free items
- Carrying a credit card
- Carrying more cash than you need
- Browsing in any store without a clear plan or budget.
- Gifts from others
- Having coupons

Things
- Newspapers
- Art/craft supplies
- Books
- Food
- Clothing
- Coupons/discount clubs
- Carrying a credit card
- Carrying more cash than you need
- Browsing in any store without a clear plan or budget

CLASS TASK: Identifying High-Risk Situations

Spend some time thinking about the things you acquire and identify some of the internal and external reasons for acquiring.

What are some of the high-risk emotions that lead to acquiring?
What are some of the high-risk stores/places that lead to acquiring?
What are some of the high-risk items that are difficult to walk away from?

Internal triggers (mood states, emotions, thoughts, physical sensations) that may lead me to acquire:

_____

_____

_____

People that may trigger my acquiring, or help me acquire:

_____

_____

_____

Places or situations that trigger acquiring for me:

_____

_____

_____

Other cues that may trigger my acquiring:

_____

_____

_____

Now that you have identified these situations as high risk, it is important that you start to stay away from them as much as possible. This will be difficult at first, but the more you practice, the easier it will be to stay away from these high-risk situations. Many people in our past classes have said that this really helped them to reduce their acquiring. We think you will find the same thing.

The next thing to consider is the difference between healthy and unhealthy acquiring.

Understanding Healthy vs. Unhealthy Acquiring

An important part of overcoming acquiring is to understand the reasons for it and to distinguish "healthy" from "unhealthy" buying and acquiring. Typical healthy and unhealthy reasons for buying or acquiring various items are outlined below.

Healthy reasons
- I have run out of the product at home.
- I have an immediate need for the item.
- It will be used to feed me and/or my family.
- It will replace something that is worn out or broken.
- I had planned to buy it before going to the store (it was on the shopping list).

Unhealthy reasons
- Because I am feeling an intense emotion and I want it to go away.
- Because it's on sale.
- Because it's free.
- Because it's visually attractive.
- To please or impress other people.
- I could use it later.
- I'll regret not getting it later.

CLASS TASK: Identifying Common Unhealthy Reasons for Acquiring

Look at the items that the class leaders have brought to class today. Is there something there that you would like to acquire? List your reasons for acquiring below. Are they healthy or unhealthy reasons? Discuss your thoughts with the class.

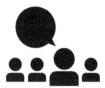

My reasons for acquiring this object:

1. _____

2. _____

3. _____

4. _____

5. _____

Learning the difference between healthy and unhealthy acquiring is important so that you can start to only acquire for "healthy" reasons.

Now let's learn about some simple guidelines that you can follow to help you to reduce your acquiring.

Guidelines for Acquiring

In order to help you to reduce your acquiring, we have come up with 10 simple guidelines. A lot of people from our previous classes have said that sticking to these guidelines really helped them to significantly reduce or eliminate their acquiring. It might be helpful to put these guidelines somewhere visible so that you are always reminded of them.

10 guidelines to reduce excessive acquiring

1. **Ditch the credit card.**   Ideally, we recommend that you cut up the credit card, give it to a trusted friend, or call the bank to freeze it. At an absolute minimum, you should leave your credit card at home when you go shopping.

2. **Avoid high-risk areas/people/things.**   Avoid the places/people/things that would normally lead you to acquire items when at all possible (discussed above). Shop infrequently and only to get what you need. Never browse, and don't enter stores just to kill time or to see what's there.

3. **Only acquire for "healthy" reasons.**   Only acquire items for the healthy reasons that we talked about – never for "unhealthy" reasons.

4. **Have a budget.**   Make a budget (i.e., make a list of the things that you need based on the healthy reasons for acquiring information) and only take the cash you need to buy those items when entering into high-risk areas. Do not carry any more cash than you need for the items you plan to buy.

5. **Use a list.**   Always use a shopping list when you leave the house and don't acquire anything that isn't on the list.

6. **Don't use a shopping cart.**   Don't use shopping carts or trolleys, unless at the grocery store. This will help you to reduce your tendency to buy extra things.

7. **Use the closest entrance/exit.**   Use the entrance/exit nearest to the store or department that you need to buy an item from. This will mean that you don't have to walk past other high-risk stores or other items that you would normally want to acquire.

8. **24-hour rule.**   If you see something that you want, but it isn't on your list, you must wait 24 hours to buy it. This will give you an opportunity to think about whether you really need it.

9. **Ride the wave of your emotions.**   Instead of buying to reduce unhelpful emotions, let these emotions decline on their own without buying something.

10. **Cancel subscriptions.**   Cancel subscriptions to newspapers, magazines, and other materials that come to your home on a regular basis.

3.   Solving Problems

We often see that people with hoarding disorder have difficulty solving many problems in their lives. Some common problems that relate to acquiring include:

- Acquiring things as gifts from friends and family
- Difficulties refusing pamphlets or free things
- Acquiring things because they might come in handy one day or might be worth money someday
- Acquiring things because you or someone else might be able to use it someday
- Acquiring things that are not in the budget
- Acquiring things that there is no room for
- Getting excessive mail
- Acquiring things just because they are on sale or appear to be a good deal
- Obtaining more object(s) in order to solve a bigger problem, e.g., "I can't sort these papers until I have files and a file cabinet."
- Acquiring things to be generous to others, or showing love by purchasing or acquiring for others

- Acquiring excessive information/paperwork because you may read/use it someday
- Acquiring more of an object because you can't find it in your home

Some common problems that can arise for people with hoarding disorder that relate to discarding include:

- Having a lot of belongings that were given to you by a family member who has now passed
- Wanting to have a garage sale but not knowing how
- Wanting to donate items rather than throw them away
- Not knowing how to ask people for help with discarding
- Not knowing how to move items to their final "home" (e.g., closet) when it's already full
- Not knowing how to have household items fixed when the house is too cluttered
- Family members who also have a problem with clutter
- Physical disabilities, poverty, or some other obstacle that makes it difficult to discard

CLASS TASK: Identifying Problems That Maintain My Clutter Problem

What are some of the main problems (mentioned above or other) that lead you to acquire items or have trouble discarding them?

1. _____
2. _____
3. _____

Learning How to Solve Problems

Effective problem solving is an important skill for everyone to learn. When we can solve problems we feel less overwhelmed by them. Learning effective problem solving is a skill like anything else and it will take time to practice. You can use problem-solving skills for any problem that occurs in your life.

There are three important steps in learning how to problem solve:

- **Step 1:** *Name the problem*
- **Step 2:** *Brainstorm solutions and consider the pros and cons of each solution*
- **Step 3:** *Select preferred solution(s)*

Let's see an example.

One of the most common problems that relates to acquiring is when people acquire items that are free from people they know. Let's practice problem solving using this example.

Step 1: Name the problem
We want to try to be as specific as we can when we identify the problem and define it in behavioral terms (your behavior). For instance, "I have too much stuff" is not specific enough, whereas "I take too many items from other people" is more specific.

Example problem: *I take too many items from other people*

Step 2: Brainstorm solutions and consider the pros and cons of each solution
At this step we want to try to come up with as many possible solutions to the problem as we can. They don't have to be good solutions, or even realistic ones at this stage. We just want to come up with a list of options. You may also like to ask trusted friends, family members, or your class leaders about possible solutions. We then want to look at the pros and cons of each solution.

1. *Stop talking to the person that is giving me the stuff*
   - *Pros:* I won't acquire as much stuff
   - *Cons:* I will be reducing my social circle even further
2. *Tell them that the stuff is causing a problem for me and ask them to stop*
   - *Pros:* It may stop the giving, and we can maintain our friendship
   - *Cons:* They will know I have a problem with clutter or may be hurt that I asked them to stop
3. *Yell at them and tell them they are trying to sabotage my efforts*
   - *Pros:* I won't get any more stuff
   - *Cons:* They may no longer want to talk to me and I will reduce my social circle even further
4. *Throw all the stuff in the trash can after they give it to me*
   - *Pros:* I can get rid of it quickly
   - *Cons:* It is hard for me to throw anything in the trash
5. *Give the stuff to someone else*
   - *Pros:* I will get rid of the thing
   - *Cons:* It is time consuming to figure out who to give it to and I may just be contributing to someone else's problem – plus I have plenty of my own stuff to get rid of
6. *Donate the stuff*
   - *Pros:* I get rid of the item
   - *Cons:* It is time consuming and I have other important things to spend my time on like getting rid of my own stuff

Step 3: Select preferred solution(s)

From the list of solutions, and after considering the pros and cons of each, it is important to choose the best option. This may not be the perfect option, but it is the option with the least amount of cons. In some cases, you may be able to select more than one solution to try.

In this example the preferred solution may be the second one:

> *Tell them that the stuff is causing a problem for me and ask them politely to stop giving me items*

CLASS TASK: Practice Problem Solving

Choose a problem that contributes to your clutter and use the problem-solving worksheet to develop a solution to this problem.

If you cannot identify a problem that leads to acquiring, you may wish to ask the class leaders for their suggestions.

Problem-Solving Worksheet

Step 1: Name the problem (in behavioral terms)

_____

Step 2: Brainstorm solutions (no matter how outrageous) and consider the pros and cons.

1. _____

2. _____

3. _____

4. _____

5. _____

6. _____

7. _____

8. _____

9. _____

10. _____

Step 3: Select preferred solution(s)

_____

4. Discarding Practice

It is important to regularly practice discarding in the class (as well as at home). In many of the classes we will put some time aside to make sure that we are practicing our discarding. You can ask the class leaders for help at this time if you need to.

Spend some time working with the class to improve your discarding. You can use the discarding flowchart to help you remember how to do this.

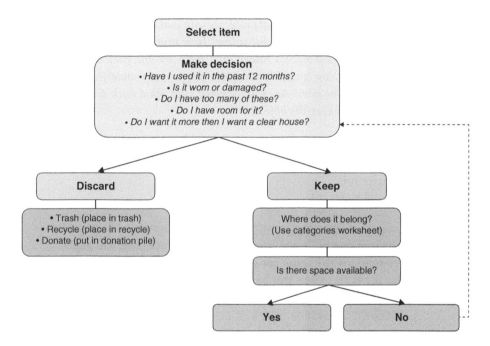

5. Bad Guy Re-evaluation

CLASS TASK: Bad Guy Evaluation

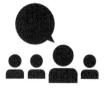

Over the past two weeks we have talked about the decision making and problem solving bad guy. Take some time to evaluate how much you think this bad guy is contributing to your acquiring behavior and difficulty discarding over the past couple weeks. Rate from 0 (not a problem for me) to 10 (a very big problem for me).

Acquiring: *How much do you think problems with decision-making and problem solving are getting in the way and are affecting your acquiring? How much do you* *notice that you are unable to weigh up the pros and cons and think through your decision when you are wanting to acquire an item?*

0 —— 1 —— 2 —— 3 —— 4 —— 5 —— 6 —— 7 —— 8 —— 9 —— 10

0 = Not a problem for me
10 = A very big problem for me

Discarding: *How much do you think that problems with making decisions and problem solving are getting in the way of your discarding? How much do you notice that you want to sift through your belongings rather than focus on one particular item and make a decision about it? How much do you notice your mind wandering, rather than making a decision about the item? Are you changing your mind back and forth about whether or not you should keep the object?*

0 —— 1 —— 2 —— 3 —— 4 —— 5 —— 6 —— 7 —— 8 —— 9 —— 10

0 = Not a problem for me
10 = A very big problem for me

How do your ratings today compare with your original ratings in Chapter 2?
    If your score came down: Congratulations – you're beating the bad guy!
    If your score remains the same (or is higher): We need to problem solve how you can practice the skills to beat this bad guy!

6.   Homework

Remember that people who do the most homework do the best at the end of the class. We recommend spending at least 1 hour a day working through your homework tasks (at least 30 minutes of this should focus exclusively on discarding).

Your homework this week is:

1. **Reread information from week 4 (including Rita's story).**
2. **Practice using the In and Out Log every day.**
3. **Practice discarding for a minimum of 30 minutes per day.**
4. **Complete weekly SMART goal.**
5. **Bring items from home to class next week.**
6. **Practice the problem-solving worksheet with a different problem related to your clutter.**
7. **Other:** _____

My SMART goal for this week:

_____

What will be my personal reward for completing my SMART goal this week?

Reward: _____

When will I give myself the reward?

Day: _____

Did I accomplish my SMART goal?   Yes   No

If no, what got in the way? _____

Rita's Story

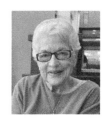

Hi everyone. I hope you have all been well over the past week.

In the class this week you talked about ways to make better decisions and resist acquiring. You also learned about a structured approach to problem solving.

I had a lot of trouble using the problem-solving skill at first. I just didn't see how it was going to be helpful. It wasn't until the next week in class when someone else talked about how helpful it had been that I decided to give it a go. I tried it out with a problem that I was having with my landlord. I was really surprised to see that there were a lot of solutions to my problem that I hadn't even considered before. I was able to make a decision about how to address the problem and so far it seems to have really helped. I'm glad that I actually gave it a go in the end!

I also used the 10 guidelines pretty regularly. There were some good ones on there that I hadn't thought of before. I found that by looking at the guidelines several times before and during a shopping trip or high-risk situation, I was better able to resist acquiring – maybe because the guidelines were fresh in my mind. Over time I learned them by heart but still needed to go over them before I left the house.

Good luck with achieving your SMART goal this week. Hopefully you are on track to receive your class reward soon! I know in my class we got a real kick out of it.

Rita.

In and Out Log – Week 4

Date	In	Out

Chapter 5/16

Intense Emotions

Part 1

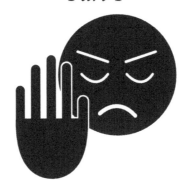

1.   Homework Review

CLASS TASK: Homework Review

We will now go around the class and discuss each person's homework and whether they have achieved their SMART goal.
   The homework tasks from last week were:

1.   **Reread information from week 4 (including Rita's story).**
2.   **Practice using the In and Out Log every day.**

CBT for Hoarding Disorder: A Group Therapy Program Workbook, First Edition. David F. Tolin, Bethany M. Wootton, Blaise L. Worden, and Christina M. Gilliam.
© 2017 John Wiley & Sons Ltd. Published 2017 by John Wiley & Sons Ltd.

3. **Practice discarding for a minimum of 30 minutes per day.**
4. **Complete weekly SMART goal.**
5. **Bring items from home to class next week.**
6. **Practice the problem-solving worksheet with a different problem related to your clutter.**
7. **Other:** _____

- Did you accomplish your SMART goal for the week? If not, how will you change things to make it more likely you will succeed this week? **Remember that the more you practice the skills, the better you will be at the end of the class!**
- Did you reward yourself? **Remember that rewards help to keep your motivation high.**

_____

_____

_____

_____

_____

Now let's learn more about intense emotions.

2. About Intense Emotions

Emotions are a normal part of life. We all experience many different emotions from time to time. Emotions can get in the way when they lead to unhelpful behaviors, such as acquiring things that we don't need or can't afford.

Intense emotions can also get in the way of discarding things we don't need or have space for. For example, some people might feel anxious, thinking that they may need the item later on. Other times, we might feel sad when attempting to discard something that has sentimental meaning attached to it. Some of us may feel guilty if we think that it's wasteful to throw things away.

In fact, avoiding discarding because of negative emotions seems to be one of the most common reasons people have hoarding disorder. Most people with hoarding disorder *want* to live a life with less clutter. They intend and plan to declutter every day. So what happens?

- We start to declutter and experience a negative emotion and stop.
- We think about decluttering, experience a negative emotion, and never get started.

- We start to declutter a specific area, experience a negative emotion, and decide to switch to a different area, jumping from one area to another, never really accomplishing anything.
- We start to declutter, experience a negative emotion, and end up "churning" – just making more piles of things rather than letting go of anything.
- We make excuses about why we can't declutter, without even being aware that we are avoiding because of an intense emotion.

CLASS TASK: Class Discussion About Intense Emotions

Do you think any of these behaviors play a role in your clutter? Are there other ways that intense emotions keep you from decluttering?

Emotions can be complex. Sometimes we can feel two or three different kinds of emotions at the same time. Sometimes it can also be hard to describe our emotions. The first step in tackling intense emotions is to learn how to identify our emotions. This can be more difficult than it sounds. But by understanding what kind of emotions we experience when acquiring or discarding, we have a better chance of coping with them in a more effective way. Some of the most common emotions include the following.

Anxiety   Anxiety is sometimes called fear. When people are anxious they tend to feel scared about something bad happening. When you feel anxious, you might notice that your heart rate speeds up, or that your breathing becomes shallow, or that you feel sweaty or clammy.

Sadness   When people feel sad or depressed they often describe feeling down and blue. They often also feel tired or fatigued and feel like they have no motivation to do anything. Sadness that is very intense can be called depression.

Anger   When people feel angry they tend to feel like they have been wronged in some way or some injustice has occurred. When people are angry they tend to feel changes in their body – they may feel hot, like their blood is boiling, they often describe tenseness in their muscles and describe clenching their fists or teeth.

Loneliness   When people feel lonely they often feel like they have no one to talk to or turn to.

Grief   When people experience grief it is often because they have lost someone or something that was very important to them. A person may have died or a relationship may have ended for other reasons.

Excitement   People may feel excitement when they are looking forward to something. They may also experience a "rush" of positive emotion.

Joy   We experience joy when we are thinking about or doing something we enjoy. Joy is also called happiness or contentment.

CLASS TASK: Identifying the Intense Emotions That Lead to Clutter

You will notice that the class leaders have some items out in the center of the table. Select an item that you would usually like to acquire. Think about what emotion(s) is causing you to want to acquire that item or think about emotions that have caused you to acquire things recently. To make things easier, listed below are some common emotions people experience when acquiring.

As I look at/touch this object, I am feeling (circle as many that apply):

Fearful	Angry	Sad	Joyful	Guilty
Anxious	Annoyed	Empty	Excited	Ashamed
Nervous	Frustrated	Lonely	Interested	Regretful
Worried	Irritated	Blue	Curious	Bored
Scared	Irked	Down	Happy	Overwhelmed
Other:				

Are there other emotions not listed on here? Add them in the empty space.

Now let's try this exercise again with discarding. As you practice discarding from your box of possessions, identify the emotions that you experience as you discard the item and after you discard it.

As I look at/touch this object and think about letting it go, I am feeling (circle as many that apply):

Fearful	Angry	Sad	Joyful	Guilty
Anxious	Annoyed	Empty	Excited	Ashamed
Nervous	Frustrated	Lonely	Interested	Regretful
Worried	Irritated	Blue	Curious	Bored
Scared	Irked	Down	Happy	Overwhelmed
Other:				

Are there other emotions not listed on here? Add them in the empty space.

After I have discarded the object I am feeling (circle as many that apply):

Fearful	Angry	Sad	Joyful	Guilty
Anxious	Annoyed	Empty	Excited	Ashamed
Nervous	Frustrated	Lonely	Interested	Regretful
Worried	Irritated	Blue	Curious	Bored
Scared	Irked	Down	Happy	Overwhelmed
Other:				

Are there other emotions not listed on here? Add them in the empty space.

3.   Tackling Intense Emotions That Lead to Acquiring

As mentioned earlier, emotions are a normal part of being human. We are not suggesting that you try to get rid of your emotions. Instead, we want you to learn how to *handle* intense emotions (positive or negative) so that they lead to helpful behaviors, rather than unhelpful behaviors, such as unnecessary acquiring or avoidance of discarding.

Often, we get in the habit of saying that a negative emotion influenced our behavior. You might say, for example, "I tried walking away from that item but I felt really anxious, so I had to go back and buy it."

But here's an alternative way to think about it: Your emotions do not control your actions. Emotions are harmless and natural. But when you have negative *beliefs* about emotions, you allow yourself to be controlled. So the *beliefs about emotions* are the problem, not the emotions themselves.

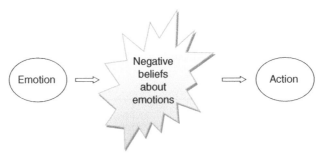

CLASS TASK: Identifying Negative
Beliefs About Emotions

Do any of these statements sound like how you think about emotions? Do these types of beliefs come up when you are trying to resist acquiring or are trying to discard things?

- I can't throw this away, I'll regret it forever.
- If I don't buy this item, I'll be upset for the rest of the day.
- I have to buy something in order to make myself feel better.
- If I throw this away, I'll be so upset that I won't be able to cope.
- Experiencing any negative emotion is bad.
- It's important to make negative emotions go away as quickly as possible.
- I'll go crazy if I keep feeling this way.

Do you have any other beliefs that might be contributing to your acquiring or difficulty discarding? List them below:

_____

_____

_____

One way to handle emotions more effectively is to view them in a different way. Rather than viewing emotions as unacceptable (it's not OK to feel negative emotions), intolerable (I can't cope or function if I feel very upset), or permanent (this bad feeling will last forever), we can think of them as what they really are: just emotions. Here are some alternative views about emotions:

- Emotions are normal and OK – even negative ones.
- Everyone experiences negative emotions from time to time.
- Emotions might not feel good, but they won't hurt me.
- Even intense emotions don't last forever.
- I don't have to act on my emotions. I can act on what's important to me.
- I CAN throw things away, even if I'm afraid that I'll regret it later.
- If I don't buy this item, I might feel upset, but I CAN cope.
- I'll feel sad for a little while if I throw this away, not forever.
- I don't have to buy something in order to feel better. The bad feeling will go away on its own, or I can do something else to cope with the bad feeling.
- All emotions will pass with time.

Can you think of other, more helpful ways of thinking about negative emotions? Write them below:

_____

_____

_____

_____

_____

4. Homework

Remember that people who do the most homework do the best at the end of the class. We recommend spending at least 1 hour a day working through your homework tasks (at least 30 minutes of this should focus exclusively on discarding).

Your homework this week is:

1. **Reread information from week 5 (including Rita's story).**
2. **Practice using the In and Out Log every day.**
3. **Practice discarding for a minimum of 30 minutes per day.**
4. **Complete weekly SMART goal.**
5. **Bring items from home to class next week.**
6. **Other:** _____

My SMART goal for this week:

_____

What will be my personal reward for completing my SMART goal this week?
Reward: _____

When will I give myself the reward?
Day: _____

Did I accomplish my SMART goal?   Yes   No
If no, what got in the way? _____

Rita's Story

Hi everyone. I learned a lot in this lesson about intense emotions and my avoidance. I could see that I did all kinds of avoiding – I avoided decluttering altogether, skipping around from room to room, and I would also make up excuses about why I couldn't discard, like my back was sore or something.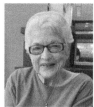

I now realize that I did all this avoiding because I was scared of feeling regret, anxiety, or sadness when I discarded what I had in front of me. It was really frustrating because it seemed like I was spending so much time trying to declutter, but never accomplishing anything. This just made me feel worse and felt like I wasn't getting anywhere in the class.

I spent some time trying to figure out what my beliefs were that related to my emotions. I never liked to experience bad emotions, but I think over time the more I tried to avoid them, the less good I was at tolerating them. It was helpful to see that I could learn to tolerate my emotions again, but I knew it would take time.

Good luck with understanding your intense emotions and what your beliefs are about them over the next week.

Rita.

In and Out Log – Week 5

Date	In	Out

Chapter 6/16

Intense Emotions

Part 2

Overview

---

1. Homework Review

CLASS TASK: Homework Review

We will now go around the class and discuss each person's homework and whether they have achieved their SMART goal.

CBT for Hoarding Disorder: A Group Therapy Program Workbook, First Edition. David F. Tolin, Bethany M. Wootton, Blaise L. Worden, and Christina M. Gilliam.
© 2017 John Wiley & Sons Ltd. Published 2017 by John Wiley & Sons Ltd.

The homework tasks from last week were:

1. **Reread information from week 5 (including Rita's story).**
2. **Practice using the In and Out Log every day.**
3. **Practice discarding for a minimum of 30 minutes per day.**
4. **Complete weekly SMART goal.**
5. **Bring items from home to class next week.**
6. **Other:** _____

- Did you accomplish your SMART goal for the week? If not, how will you change things to make it more likely you will succeed this week? **Remember that the more you practice the skills, the better you will be at the end of the class!**
- Did you reward yourself? **Remember that rewards help to keep your motivation high.**

_____

_____

_____

_____

_____

Now let's learn more about dealing with intense emotions.

2.   Tackling Intense Emotions That Get in the Way of Discarding

Accepting Our Emotions and Being Our Own Boss

Last week we talked a lot about intense emotions and how they can make a clutter problem worse. In this class we want to talk more about other ways to respond to emotions. Rather than acting on our emotions by acquiring or avoiding discarding, we suggest *accepting* our emotions instead.

Let's learn more about what this means.

Learning to accept emotions involves three steps.

Step 1: Just observe
The first step in accepting our emotions is to *observe* and *describe* what we are experiencing. At this point, don't make judgments about the emotions, thoughts, sensations, or the situation. Simply notice, observe, and describe. In other words,

the goal is to become *aware* of our emotions without trying to change them or get rid of them. This is probably quite different than what you would normally do when you experience intense emotions (positive or negative), so it'll take some practice.

Step 2: Know what's important to you and be your own boss
The next step in handling intense emotions is to act in a way that is consistent with *your* values and goals, rather than allowing your emotions to be your boss. It's very natural to be tempted to act based on our emotions. For example, when we are sad, we may have the urge to isolate ourselves and stay in bed. When we are feeling anxious, we have the urge to avoid whatever it is that makes us feel anxious, including discarding. When we are excited about an object, we may have the urge to acquire it. But if we act on these urges, who's the boss? You, or your emotions?

Below are some examples of using the Be Your Own Boss technique. This example involves someone who has a SMART goal that involves decluttering their bedroom.

Situation	Emotions as boss	Me as boss
Thinking about decluttering my bedroom. I feel overwhelmed.	Don't know where to start so I never get started	Make a step-by-step list of how to tackle the bedroom, breaking it into easier chunks
Trying to discard sentimental objects. It makes me feel sad.	Stop decluttering for the day	Practice "observing" my emotions, think of other ways to remember fond memories, then return to decluttering
Decluttering the top of my bed, so I can sleep on it – I can feel myself getting frustrated.	Switch to decluttering a different room	Set a timer for 10 minutes to allow myself a break when I get too frustrated, then return to decluttering the bed
Decluttering a pile of clothes I haven't worn in years. I feel anxious and can't decide what to keep.	Can't decide what to keep so I just end up keeping everything	Practice "observing" my emotions. Focus on my goals, rather than keeping clothes just because of my anxiety

We will review your values more when we talk about motivation in a later chapter. However, for now, please write down 2–3 important values and goals that motivate your decluttering right now, so that you know what values should be guiding you. Some examples of goals might be "to provide a safe environment for my kids/grand-kids" or "to decrease arguments with my spouse/partner."

1. _____

2. _____

3. _____

Step3: Ride the wave

The final (and possibly the most difficult) step is to *act* in line with your goals, rather than your emotions. This means doing what is important to you, *even* if that means you will feel a negative emotion (e.g., sad, anxious, regretful).

We call our strategy "riding the wave." Imagine a surfer on top of a wave. The wave is very powerful, yet the surfer is able to travel on top of it, rather than falling into it and being tossed around.

Dealing with uncomfortable emotions can be a bit like surfing. Your emotions are powerful, and they can easily toss you around if you let them. But you can ride on top of your emotions. The trick is to *tolerate* your emotions, rather than try to struggle against them. When you stop trying to control or avoid your feelings, you'll find that you can dedicate more energy and time to acting in a way that is consistent with your values. Riding the wave means being brave and doing what you need to do to achieve your goals. Emotions are like waves – they go up and down. Just like a surfer, once you ride the wave, a period of calm is often the result.

CLASS TASK: Being Your Own Boss: Acquiring

Select an item from the center of the table that you are tempted to acquire. As you hold the object, practice being aware of your emotions. Describe the object, memories, and ideas associated with the object. Practice as many times as you can.

_____

_____

_____

Next, let's practice *being your own boss*, rather than your emotions being your boss. Use the worksheet below. Another example is also provided below.

Example: Resisting acquiring a hardcover book

Describe and Observe	Emotions as boss	Me as boss
"Hard surface, heavy. Love the feeling of a real book in my hands. Memories of reading, feeling content, when I was a kid. This looks like a great book – I should take it. I still love reading. I'll regret it later if I don't take it.	Take the book home.	Resist the urge to acquire the book. Practice observing and riding the wave. Think of how resisting the urge is helping me to accomplish my SMART goal. Remind myself that this feeling of regret won't last forever.

My top goals and values:

_____

_____

Describe and Observe	Emotions as boss	Me as boss

CLASS TASK: Being Your Own Boss: Discarding

Now let's try the same exercise, but with discarding. As you practice your discarding try being aware of your emotions. Describe the object, memories, and ideas associated with the object. What are you feeling and thinking as you think about discarding this object? Use the worksheet below.

Example: Discarding a cute flower pot

Describe and Observe	Emotions as boss	Me as boss
"Green, small, has an adorable frog face on it. Looking at it makes me feel happy – I'm thinking about the different flowers I can plant in it. It'll be wasteful to throw this out – nothing is wrong with it.	Keep the flower pot. Put it back where it was – in a pile in my bedroom, intending to plant flowers in it (but I haven't done it for the past 10 years).	Discard the flower pot. Remind myself that I can be brave and let it go, even though I'm afraid I'll regret it later. Picture a clean bedroom where I can relax.

My top goals and values:

_____

_____

Describe and Observe	Emotions as boss	Me as boss

Recognizing When Emotions Are Taking Over

One of the biggest challenges of "being your own boss" is knowing when you are in charge and when you are not. Often when our emotions take over we start to avoid discarding. Sometimes knowing when you're in charge and when you're not can be obvious – there might be times when you *know* you are avoiding discarding because of a negative emotion. But it's probably just as likely that you avoid discarding without knowing it! How often do any of the following happen?

- You don't get around to discarding because you're too busy; too much is going on.
- You don't get around to discarding because your family gets in the way.
- You don't discard because you don't have the proper materials yet (e.g., boxes, file cabinet).
- You don't discard because you're too tired.
- Problems keep coming up that get in the way.
- You plan to do it after you get everything else done, and then it's too late.
- You only discard the "lower hanging fruit" – meaning you discard only the easiest stuff, never making any real progress.
- You can't discard right now because you're not in the mood.

Can you think of other examples when we might not recognize we're avoiding discarding?

_____

_____

_____

Have you ever heard someone come up with multiple reasons why they didn't get around to doing something, even if they say it's really important? Then that person is probably letting their emotions be the boss without knowing it.

In order to know when your emotions are taking over, ask yourself these questions several times a day:

- Am I making a bunch of excuses as to why I haven't been discarding? Even if they seem like good reasons?
- Have I discarded anything at all today?
- Have I discarded what I need to discard in order to reach my SMART goal by the end of the week?
- Have I saved an object *even after* I've come to the conclusion that it's probably best to let it go?

Other signs that I am letting emotions be the boss:

_____

_____

_____

Once you realize that you've been letting your emotions be your boss, you know what to do! Use the three steps you just learned in order to make sure that you are being your own boss.

3.   Bad Guy Re-evaluation

CLASS TASK: Bad Guy Re-evaluation

Over the past two weeks we have talked about the intense emotions bad guy. Take some time to evaluate how much you think this bad guy has been contributing to your acquiring behavior and difficulty discarding over the past couple weeks. Rate from 0 (not a problem for me) to 10 (a very big problem for me).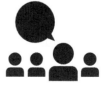

Acquiring: What kinds of emotions are you feeling when you acquire something? Interested? Excited? What kinds of emotions do you think you will experience if you don't obtain this object? Guilty? Sad? Bored? How much are these intense emotions contributing to your acquiring behavior?

0 —— 1 —— 2 —— 3 —— 4 —— 5 —— 6 —— 7 —— 8 —— 9 —— 10

0 = Not a problem for me
10 = A very big problem for me

Discarding: *What kinds of emotions are you feeling when you are discarding? What emotions do you think you will feel after you discard the object? Sadness? Grief? Anger? Frustration? Anxiety? Guilt? How much are these emotions getting in the way of you being able to discard as much as you would like to?*

0 —— 1 —— 2 —— 3 —— 4 —— 5 —— 6 —— 7 —— 8 —— 9 —— 10

0 = Not a problem for me
10 = A very big problem for me

How do your ratings today compare with your original ratings in Chapter 2?

If your score came down: Congratulations – you're beating the bad guy!

If your score remains the same (or is higher): We need to problem solve how you can practice the skills to beat this bad guy!

4.   Homework

Remember that people who do the most homework do the best at the end of the class. We recommend spending at least 1 hour a day working through your homework tasks.

Your homework this week is:

1.   **Reread information from week 6 (including Rita's story).**
2.   **Practice using the In and Out Log every day.**
3.   **Practice discarding for a minimum of 30 minutes per day.**
4.   **Complete weekly SMART goal.**
5.   **Bring items from home to class next week.**
6.   **Other:** _____

My SMART goal for this week:
_____

What will be my personal reward for completing my SMART goal this week?
Reward: _____

When will I give myself the reward?
Day: _____

Did I accomplish my SMART goal?   Yes   No
If no, what got in the way? _____

Rita's Story

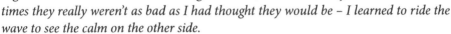

Over the past two weeks I sure did learn a lot about my intense emotions and how they contribute to my clutter problem.

The most important thing that I learned was that to feel less anxious and less upset in the long term, I had to feel a bit of discomfort up front. It was like short-term pain for long-term gain!

After a few weeks of practicing I really learned that I can tolerate negative emotions more than I thought I could, and that many times they really weren't as bad as I had thought they would be – I learned to ride the wave to see the calm on the other side.

Just like with all the skills in this class, learning to "accept" my emotions took a lot of practice. Reminding myself of my SMART goal and values – what's important to me – every single day helped me to act in ways that were helpful rather than acting on my emotions. It wasn't always easy but I could see that the more I practiced, the more I improved.

Good luck this week. Next week you will learn about how unhelpful thoughts contribute to your clutter.

Rita.

In and Out Log – Week 6

Date	In	Out

Chapter 7/16

Unhelpful Thinking

Part 1

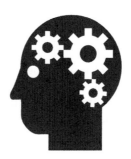

1.   Homework Review

CLASS TASK: Homework Review

We will now go around the class and discuss each person's homework and whether they have achieved their SMART goal.

CBT for Hoarding Disorder: A Group Therapy Program Workbook, First Edition. David F. Tolin, Bethany M. Wootton, Blaise L. Worden, and Christina M. Gilliam.
© 2017 John Wiley & Sons Ltd. Published 2017 by John Wiley & Sons Ltd.

The homework tasks from last week were:

1. **Reread information from week 6 (including Rita's story).**
2. **Practice using the In and Out Log every day.**
3. **Practice discarding for a minimum of 30 minutes per day.**
4. **Complete weekly SMART goal.**
5. **Bring items from home to class next week.**
6. **Other:** _____

- Did you accomplish your SMART goal for the week? If not, how will you change things to make it more likely you will succeed this week? **Remember that the more you practice the skills, the better you will be at the end of the class!**
- Did you reward yourself? **Remember that rewards help to keep your motivation high.**

_____
_____
_____
_____
_____

This week we will learn more about how unhelpful thinking can contribute to acquiring and difficulty discarding.

2.   How Thoughts Influence Emotions

As we discussed previously, the way we think about things determines how we feel about them, and as we learned in Chapters 5 and 6, our emotions can really affect our behavior.

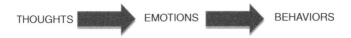

THOUGHTS ➤ EMOTIONS ➤ BEHAVIORS

Let's look at some examples of how the way someone thinks can affect their emotions and behaviors.

Imagine you are at the supermarket and you are waiting to be served. The cashier walks away before serving you.

You may think about this in a number of different ways.

If you thought...	You would probably feel...
"She probably needed to do something important and will be back in a minute."	Okay
"How dare she walk away before serving me! Who does she think she is?"	Angry
"She probably didn't serve me because she thinks I'm a loser."	Sad

So even in the same situation a person can have different thoughts about it, which leads to a different emotional response. That's because the way we *think* about the situation, not the situation itself, determines how we feel about it.

Let's try another example.

CLASS TASK: Identifying How Thoughts Lead to Emotions

Let's imagine that you were trying to clear some items in your home.

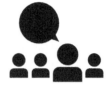

If you thought...	You would probably feel...
"Why bother trying? I'll never be able to get through it all."	
"If I throw this away I'll lose something important."	
"I have many of these items, I don't need more than one."	
"I'm really making some good progress on getting through this clutter."	

3. Identifying Unhelpful Thoughts

Common Unhelpful Thoughts in People with Hoarding Disorder

Often our thoughts can be unhelpful and people with hoarding disorder tend to have many of the same sorts of unhelpful thoughts. Some common thoughts that have come up in our past classes include the following.

See if you can identify with any of the following common thoughts:

Thoughts about responsibility
- It is my responsibility to make sure things get disposed of properly.
- I have to make sure everything goes to a "good home."
- If someone else can use it, I'm responsible for hanging on to it.
- I will disappoint someone if I get rid of it.

Thoughts about usefulness
- I need to keep it or acquire it because I'll be able to use it one day.
- I will be able to fix it one day.
- Someone will be able to use this eventually.
- I have to get this for my friend/family member because he or she could really use it/benefit from this information.

Thoughts about objects being part of your identity
- Without my possessions I would be nothing.
- These things are part of who I am.
- I need to acquire or hang on to these things so that I can be an artist/craftsperson/etc.
- I'm clever if I can find a bargain.
- A good parent/sister/brother/friend would keep this item – how can you throw away something from/made by someone you love?

Thoughts about attachment
- I need to acquire or keep the objects because they serve as reminders of important times in my life.
- My things feel like my friends.
- I have to acquire or keep this object because I don't want to make it sad.
- I'll miss the item too much.

Thoughts about value
- I paid for it, so I can't throw it away because that would be flushing money down the drain.
- I can't throw anything away that has value.
- It's mine, so it's valuable.
- If it's on sale, it makes financial sense to buy it.
- I should hang onto this item because it is worth money.
- I don't have much money; therefore, I need to save everything.

Thoughts about wastefulness
- It's wasteful to throw things away that can still be used.
- Wasteful people are horrible.
- I would be stupid to pass up a deal this great.
- I would be wasting money if I didn't purchase this now.

Thoughts about memory function
- I need to keep information close by, otherwise I will forget it.
- I need to be able to see all of my things.
- If I put this away, I'll forget it.
- I'll forget the memories that are associated with the item.

Thoughts about anticipating emotion
- I can't throw things away because I will be too sad.
- I'm so stressed out; going shopping will make me feel better.
- If I throw this away or pass this up, I'll regret it forever.

- If I become upset, I'll never get over it.
- This item is so beautiful, it will make me happy whenever I see it.

Pessimistic thoughts
- There's too much stuff – I'll never be able to get rid of it all.
- I'm not making as much progress as I'd like. Why bother at all?
- I've already spent more than I planned; I might as well buy these extra things.
- I won't be able to control my spending this weekend.

Now let's start to identify some of the unhelpful thoughts that come up for you when discarding.

TASK: Identifying Unhelpful Thoughts That Lead to Difficulty Discarding

Start working through your box of items that you brought from home. As you are working through your discarding, try to identify some of the thoughts going through your mind that make you want to keep items:

1. _____
2. _____
3. _____
4. _____
5. _____

Now let's identify some of the thoughts that lead to acquiring. Choose an item from the class leaders' belongings that you would normally like to acquire. As you look at the item and handle the item, take note of the thoughts that go through your mind when you think about acquiring the object, and when you think about leaving it behind.

1. _____
2. _____
3. _____
4. _____
5. _____

What type of beliefs did you notice come up the most?

1. _____
2. _____
3. _____
4. _____
5. _____

4.   Homework

Remember that people who do the most homework do the best at the end of the class. We recommend spending at least 1 hour a day working through your homework tasks.

Your homework this week is:

1. **Reread information from week 7 (including Rita's story).**
2. **Practice using the In and Out Log every day.**
3. **Practice discarding for a minimum of 30 minutes per day.**
4. **Bring items from home to class next week.**
5. **Take photos of your progress for your mid-treatment review.**
6. **Complete weekly SMART goal.**
7. **Other:** _____

My SMART goal for this week:
_____

What will be my personal reward for completing my SMART goal this week?
Reward: _____

When will I give myself the reward?
Day: _____

Did I accomplish my SMART goal?   Yes   No
If no, what got in the way? _____

Rita's Story

Hi everyone. I hope that you have been working hard on reducing your clutter.

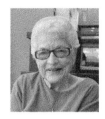

This class helped me to notice a lot of my unhelpful thoughts. I'd never noticed how many unhelpful thoughts I was having. One of the most common unhelpful thoughts that I could identify in myself that related to acquiring was "I must buy things at the sale price." I would get really angry with myself if I didn't get things at sale price. I remember one time an item was on sale but I didn't have enough money, and then when I went back to get it the item was gone. I felt angry for days!

I was also able to identify thoughts that contributed to me having trouble throwing things away, especially the thoughts about usefulness (because I consider myself to be quite the fix-it person). I realized that I had thoughts like "I can fix it one day" fairly often when I was trying to discard. It was so hard to think about getting rid of some of my items, especially since I knew they would be worth money if I fixed them, and I felt like getting rid of them was just like throwing money down the drain.

I was looking forward to starting to work on reducing some of these unhelpful thoughts. I could see how they were really affecting my mood and made me act in a way that was not in line with my goals and values. I was hoping that I would be able to learn some skills to reduce my unhelpful thinking.

Good luck this week. Next week you will learn more about challenging these unhelpful thoughts.

Rita.

In and Out Log – Week 7

Date	In	Out

Chapter 8/16

Unhelpful Thinking

Part 2

1.   Homework Review

CLASS TASK: Homework Review

We will now go around the class and discuss each person's homework and whether they have achieved their SMART goal.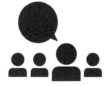
   The homework tasks from last week were:

CBT for Hoarding Disorder: A Group Therapy Program Workbook, First Edition. David F. Tolin,
Bethany M. Wootton, Blaise L. Worden, and Christina M. Gilliam.
© 2017 John Wiley & Sons Ltd. Published 2017 by John Wiley & Sons Ltd.

1. Reread information from week 7 (including Rita's story).
2. Practice using the In and Out Log every day.
3. Practice discarding for a minimum of 30 minutes per day.
4. Bring items from home to class next week.
5. Take photos of your progress for your mid-treatment review.
6. Complete weekly SMART goal.
7. Other: _____

- Did you accomplish your SMART goal for the week? If not, how will you change things to make it more likely you will succeed this week? **Remember that the more you practice the skills, the better you will be at the end of the class!**
- Did you reward yourself? **Remember that rewards help to keep your motivation high.**

_____
_____
_____
_____
_____

This week we will learn more about unhelpful thinking and how to overcome this bad guy.

2.   Tackling Unhelpful Thoughts

In the last chapter we talked a lot about identifying our unhelpful thoughts. We will continue to talk about how to tackle this bad guy in this chapter.

In this chapter we will teach you two skills to tackle the unhelpful thinking bad guy. Different skills will work for different kinds of thoughts. We will teach you how to:

- **Question the thoughts**
- **Act as you would advise a friend**

These skills can be used to target both acquiring and saving. The first skill we will teach you is to question your thoughts.

Question the Thoughts

Often people think that because they think something, it makes it true or significant – but thoughts are just thoughts. One important skill is to learn to question the unhelpful thoughts. Many people have told us that the following questions are essential to ask themselves when they are in a situation where they want to acquire something or when they have trouble throwing things away.

- *In my ideal home, is there a place for this object? When I imagine my ideal home, where does this object go?*
- *If I don't save this item or acquire this item, will anything bad happen to me?*
- *Is this item in good working order?*
- *Do I have a specific plan to use this item within the next 12 months?*
- *Would someone without a hoarding problem keep or take this item into their home?*
- *Do I have more of these than I need?*
- *Will saving this actually make me financially better off?*
- *Would I be able to get the item (or information) again in the future?*
- *Does having this thing mean more to me than having a clear house?*

CLASS TASK: Practice Questioning Your Thoughts: Acquiring

You will notice that the class leaders have some belongings that may normally be things that you would like to acquire. Please identify at least one item that you would like to take home. Once you have identified one item, try to start testing your thoughts. Pay attention to the questions that are enclosed in a box. If you answer the questions honestly and there are more  "boxed" than "unboxed" responses circled, then it is likely that you do not need the item and that it is contributing to your problem with clutter.

Item: _____

- *If I don't acquire this item will anything bad happen to me?*   YES   NO
- *Is this item in good working order?*   YES   NO
- *Do I have a specific plan to use this item within the next 12 months?*   YES   NO
- *Would someone without a hoarding problem take this item into their home?*   YES   NO
- *Do I have more of these than I need?*   YES   NO
- *Would I be able to get the item (or information) again in the future?*   YES   NO
- *Does having this thing mean more to me than having a clear house?*   YES   NO

Let's try another example, this time focusing on discarding.

CLASS TASK: Practice Questioning Your Thoughts: Discarding

Now let's start using these questions to help you question your thoughts related to discarding. As you are discarding items from your box of belongings, ask yourself the following questions:

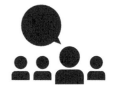

Item: _____

- *When I imagine my **ideal home**, is there a place I can see this object/where this object belongs?*   YES   NO

- *If I don't save this item, will anything bad happen to me?*   YES   NO

- *Is this item in good working order?*   YES   NO

- *Do I have a specific plan to use this item within the next 12 months?*   YES   NO

- *Would someone without a hoarding problem keep this item?*   YES   NO

- *Will saving this actually make me financially better off?*   YES   NO

- *Do I have more of these than I need?*   YES   NO

- *Would I be able to get the item (or information) again in the future?*   YES   NO

- *Does having this thing mean more to me than having a clear house?*   YES   NO

What Would You Say to a Friend?

We often respond to ourselves in a much more negative fashion than we would to other people we care about, such as friends and relatives. See the examples below for ways in which someone responds more harshly to themselves than to a friend.

Situation	What you say to yourself...	What you say to a friend...
Acquiring a pen from the bank	*I'm so stupid for acquiring that.*	*Don't beat yourself up – just try to stay on top of it next time.*
Starting discarding session	*I'll never get through all of this, so why bother?*	*It will take time, but you'll get there. Just take it a bit at a time.*
Seeing an item at a thrift store that you like	*That is such a great deal, I should buy a few of them.*	*You have been doing a great job lately not acquiring things you don't need. Are you sure you absolutely need this?*
Looking around cluttered home	*I'm such a loser for letting things get this bad.*	*Things are not as you want them to be, but with some hard work you can have your house looking the way you want it to look.*

Another important way to reduce your unhelpful thinking is to start responding to yourself as you would to a friend. Ask yourself what advice you would give to a friend in the same situation.

This task might be useful for you if you can identify any of the following kinds of thoughts:

- **Thoughts about responsibility**
- **Thoughts about usefulness**
- **Thoughts about objects being part of your identity**
- **Thoughts about value**
- **Thoughts about wastefulness**
- **Pessimistic thoughts**

CLASS TASK: How Would I Advise a Friend?

Identify a situation(s) and unhelpful thought(s) that you have been having and think about how you would respond to a friend in the same situation. Is your response the same as to yourself or is it different? How can you be kinder to yourself and respond as you would to a friend?

Situation	What you say to yourself...	What you say to a friend...

3. Bad Guy Re-evaluation

CLASS TASK: Bad Guy Re-evaluation

Over the past two weeks we have talked about the unhelpful thinking bad guy. Take some time to evaluate how much you think this bad guy is contributing to your acquiring behavior and difficulty discarding over the past couple weeks. Rate from 0 (not a problem for me) to 10 (a very big problem for me).

Acquiring: *When you are faced with a situation where you want to acquire, what is going through your mind? How much are you experiencing unhelpful thoughts? Are you thinking that you might have a good use for the item? Are you thinking that you shouldn't pass up such a great deal?*

0 —— 1 —— 2 —— 3 —— 4 —— 5 —— 6 —— 7 —— 8 —— 9 —— 10

0 = Not a problem for me
10 = A very big problem for me

Discarding: *When you are discarding, what is going through your mind? How much are you experiencing unhelpful thoughts? Are you thinking the item will be useful? Or that you're being wasteful? Or that you could give the item to a friend?*

0 —— 1 —— 2 —— 3 —— 4 —— 5 —— 6 —— 7 —— 8 —— 9 —— 10

0 = Not a problem for me
10 = A very big problem for me

How do your ratings today compare with your original ratings from Chapter 2?
   If your score came down: Congratulations – you're beating the bad guy!
   If your score remains the same (or is higher): We need to problem solve how you can practice the skills to beat this bad guy!

4. Homework

Remember that people who do the most homework do the best at the end of the class. We recommend spending at least 1 hour a day working through your homework tasks.

Your homework this week is:

1. **Reread information from week 8 (including Rita's story).**
2. **Practice using the In and Out Log every day.**
3. **Practice discarding for a minimum of 30 minutes per day.**
4. **Bring items from home to class next week.**
5. **Complete weekly SMART goal.**
6. **Other**: _____

My SMART goal for this week:

_____

What will be my personal reward for completing my SMART goal this week?
Reward: _____

When will I give myself the reward?
Day: _____

Did I accomplish my SMART goal?   Yes   No
If no, what got in the way? _____

Rita's Story

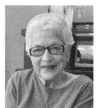

Hi everyone. Congratulations on getting this far – you are now over halfway through the Declutter Class. You should be really proud of yourself for getting this far. I know from experience that it probably hasn't been easy for you. If you are like me, you will still find that you have a lot more to learn. I think that the second part of the class really helped me to make the most gains.

In this class you talked more about problematic thoughts. When I completed the class all the class members realized that we had a lot of unhelpful thoughts, but we noticed that we all had different kinds of unhelpful thoughts and found that the different exercises were more helpful for some people than others. We all found at least one thought-challenging exercise that helped us to tackle this bad guy, though.

Even though I have a lot of thoughts about usefulness, like I need to "fix it," and thoughts about wastefulness, like "it's bad to waste things," this class helped me to realize that it wasn't worth it – that I didn't have the time to fix things, that they had been sitting around for years, and keeping them wasn't worth the clutter in my home!

I used the worksheets from this class pretty regularly. At first I would have to look at the worksheet and go through question by question, but now the questions are in my head. It took many weeks of practice to get to this point.

Good luck with your homework tasks this week. Remember that the class is counting on you to help them all reach their reward. All the best.

Rita.

In and Out Log – Week 8

Date	In	Out

Chapter 9/16

Waxing and Waning Motivation

Part 1

1. Homework Review

CLASS TASK: Homework Review

We will now go around the class and discuss each person's homework and whether they have achieved their SMART goal.

CBT for Hoarding Disorder: A Group Therapy Program Workbook, First Edition. David F. Tolin,
Bethany M. Wootton, Blaise L. Worden, and Christina M. Gilliam.
© 2017 John Wiley & Sons Ltd. Published 2017 by John Wiley & Sons Ltd.

The homework tasks from last week were:

1. **Reread information from week 8 (including Rita's story).**
2. **Practice using the In and Out Log every day.**
3. **Practice discarding for a minimum of 30 minutes per day.**
4. **Bring items from home to class next week.**
5. **Complete weekly SMART goal.**
6. **Other:** _____

- Did you accomplish your SMART goal for the week? If not, how will you change things to make it more likely you will succeed this week? **Remember that the more you practice the skills, the better you will be at the end of the class!**
- Did you reward yourself? **Remember that rewards help to keep your motivation high.**

_____
_____
_____
_____
_____

This week we will talk about ways to improve motivation.

2. Improving Motivation

The final bad guy that we will focus on in the Declutter Class is motivation. We often find that motivation tends to go up and down over the 16 weeks of the class. Often people start off very motivated, but then get less motivated over time. Most likely you will also notice that your motivation goes up and down after you finish the class.

We want you to be able to use the skills that we discuss over the next two weeks to help improve your motivation both during the class and after the class ends.

We have a number of tasks to help you increase your motivation to reduce your acquiring and improve your discarding. The skills we will learn over the next two weeks are:

- **Understanding the pros and cons of continuing your efforts**
- **Focusing on goals and values**
- **Using your imagination to see the change that is possible in your home**

Let's get started.

The Pros and Cons of Continuing Your Efforts

Often people say that there are both good and bad things about changing their behavior. An important way to increase your motivation is to consider the pros and cons of your current behavior (including discarding and nonacquiring). We can think about both the short- and long-term pros and cons of change in these areas.

CLASS TASK: Identifying Pros and Cons of Continuing Your Effort

Spend some time thinking about the good things and bad things about making changes to your behavior. Complete the following worksheet and discuss your findings with the class. Other class members might be able to identify some cons that you hadn't considered before.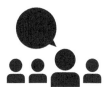

Pros and cons: example

SHORT TERM	
Advantages (Pros) of Discarding and Not Acquiring	Disadvantages (Cons) of Discarding and Not Acquiring
• *I'll be able to sleep on my bed more comfortably* • *I'll be able to eat at the kitchen table* • *I'll be able to cook and wash dishes more easily* • *I'll be able to get my dishwasher fixed* • *I'll be able to clean more easily* • *My kids will be happy with me; less arguments with them about my house/clutter* • *I'll feel better about myself*	• *I might throw something away that I regret later* • *I might miss out on a great sale that I regret later* • *I might need something that I throw out* • *It's going to take a lot of work to declutter*
LONG TERM	
Advantages (Pros) of Discarding and Not Acquiring	Disadvantages (Cons) of Discarding and Not Acquiring
• *I'll be able to invite my grandkids over to play* • *I'll be able to have friends over; socialize more* • *I won't have to worry about something breaking and being too embarrassed to have a repairman come to fix it* • *I'll be able to find things easily, spend less time looking for things* • *I might save money from not having to buy something I already have but just can't find* • *My asthma will be less problematic (easier to clean the house to keep it less dusty)*	• *I'll miss the thrill/excitement of tag sales and bargain shopping* • *I might miss out on interesting info and have less to talk about with others*

Pros and Cons of Discarding and Not Acquiring Worksheet

SHORT TERM	
Advantages (Pros) of Continuing to Work on Decluttering	Disadvantages (Cons) of Continuing to Work on Decluttering
LONG TERM	
Advantages (Pros) of Continuing to Work on Decluttering	Disadvantages (Cons) of Continuing to Work on Decluttering

Now let's talk about how focusing on our goals and values can help us reduce clutter.

3. Acting on Your Top Goals and Values

Focusing on Goals and Values

We find that often people say that they value having a clear home. However, their actions do not support this because they continue to acquire items that contribute to the clutter in their home or they fail to make the behavioral changes required to clear the clutter in their home. An important part of overcoming clutter is to think about what your goals and values are for your life and whether your actions or behaviors are in line with these goals.

In order to understand if your behaviors are in line with your goals and values, we need to find out exactly what is important to you. These can be some tough questions to answer, but it is essential to think about them so that you can tell if your behaviors are consistent with your goals and values. We can have goals in many aspects of our lives. It is important that you think about what you actually value, not what you think other people think you should value.

CLASS TASK: Identifying My Life Goals and Values

Discuss with the class and answer the following questions to help you to understand what your life goals and values are.

Relationships   What's important to you about your relationships? This can include romantic relationships, friends, or family. (Examples: improve my relationship with my children, reconnect with old friends)

1. _____

2. _____

3. _____

Personal well-being   What's important to you when it comes to your personal well-being? This can include things like your health (mental and physical), spirituality, learning and education, or hobbies. (Examples: manage my diabetes better, start attending religious service, take a photography class)

1. _____

2. _____

3. _____

Career and finances   What's important to you in your career and financial future? (Examples: find a full-time job, pay off credit card debt)

1. _____
2. _____
3. _____

Now that you have defined your values, we want to know which values are the most important to you.

From your list above, what are your top 3 values?

1. _____
2. _____
3. _____

CLASS TASK: Are My Life Goals Consistent with My Acquiring and Discarding Behaviors?

Now that you have had a chance to consider your life goals and values, it is important to start to practice considering these life goals when you are in a situation when you may acquire.

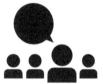

Look at the items that the class leaders brought into the session today. Choose an item that you would like to acquire. Then work through the worksheet to identify whether acquiring the item is consistent with your life goals and values. An example is provided first.

Life Goals and Values Worksheet: Example

Item that I am considering acquiring: *New wireless printer (on sale)*

What are my most important life goals and values?

1. *Have a good relationship with my kids and grandkids*
2. *Take care of my health, especially my diabetes*
3. *Get my finances in order – pay off high interest loan debts/credit cards*

Would acquiring this item be consistent with my life goals and values?   Yes/ No

What will be the consequence of acquiring this item?

1. *It'll add to the clutter, taking me away from my goal of cleaning up enough to have my grandkids visit*
2. *My kids will be upset with me; I already have 3 printers that I don't use*
3. *Add to my credit card debt, even if it's on sale*

What do I need to do in order to be consistent with my goals and values in this situation?

Don't buy it; just use the printers I already have. I just need to make space to use it

Life Goals and Values Worksheet

Item that I am considering acquiring: _____

What are my most important life goals and values?

1. _____
2. _____
3. _____

Would acquiring this item be consistent with my life goals and values?   Yes / No

What will be the consequence of acquiring this item?

1. _____
2. _____
3. _____
4. _____
5. _____

What do I need to do in order to be consistent with my goals and values in this situation?

_____

_____

_____

_____

Now let's focus on discarding. As you are working through discarding the items that you brought from home, think about whether your behavior is consistent with your life goals and values. If you find there is an item that you are not able to discard, then work through the following worksheet.

Item that I am considering discarding: _____

What are my most important life goals and values?

1. _____
2. _____
3. _____

Would discarding this item be consistent with my life goals and values?   Yes/No

What will be the benefits of discarding this item?

1. _____
2. _____
3. _____
4. _____
5. _____

What do I need to do in order to be consistent with my goals and values in this situation?

_____
_____
_____
_____

4.   Homework

Remember that people who do the most homework do the best at the end of the class. We recommend spending at least 1 hour a day working through your homework tasks.

Your homework this week is:

1.   Reread information from week 9 (including Rita's story).
2.   Practice using the In and Out Log every day.
3.   Practice discarding for a minimum of 30 minutes per day.
4.   Complete weekly SMART goal.
5.   Bring items from home to class next week.
6.   Other: _____

My SMART goal for this week:
_____

What will be my personal reward for completing my SMART goal this week?
Reward: _____

When will I give myself the reward?
Day: _____

Did I accomplish my SMART goal?   Yes   No
If no, what got in the way? _____

Rita's Story

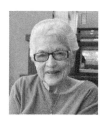

I hope you have had a good week and that you are starting to really understand and tackle your clutter problem. In this class you learned how to boost motivation, which often tends to go up and down over time.

The most important part of this class for me was considering my life goals. This was not something that I had really considered before. When I was thinking it through, I realized that I wanted people to say nice things about me when I die, but I wasn't sure that they would. I mean, my clutter had really affected my relationships with my friends and family and I wasn't sure anyone would say anything nice about me. I didn't want to be the woman with all the junk that someone else had to clean up after I died. This made me really motivated to not only decrease my acquiring, but also get a move on with my decluttering.

I found that using the "Life goals and values worksheet" helped when I was faced with a situation where I wanted to acquire something. I would first consider whether bringing the item home would be consistent with my values – and generally it wasn't. So most of the time I didn't take it home. This requires a lot of will power, but I was able to improve with time and I noticed that I really reduced my acquiring over the next few weeks.

Good luck with the second motivational lesson next week.

Rita.

In and Out Log – Week 9

Date	In	Out

Chapter 10/16

Waxing and Waning Motivation
Part 2

Overview

---

1.   Homework Review

CLASS TASK: Homework Review

We will now go around the class and discuss each person's homework and whether they have achieved their SMART goal.

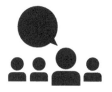

CBT for Hoarding Disorder: A Group Therapy Program Workbook, First Edition. David F. Tolin, Bethany M. Wootton, Blaise L. Worden, and Christina M. Gilliam.
© 2017 John Wiley & Sons Ltd. Published 2017 by John Wiley & Sons Ltd.

The homework tasks from last week were:

1. **Reread information from week 9 (including Rita's story).**
2. **Practice using the In and Out Log every day.**
3. **Practice discarding for a minimum of 30 minutes per day.**
4. **Complete weekly SMART goal.**
5. **Bring items from home to class next week.**
6. **Other:** _____

- Did you accomplish your SMART goal for the week? If not, how will you change things to make it more likely you will succeed this week? **Remember that the more you practice the skills, the better you will be at the end of the class!**
- Did you reward yourself? **Remember that rewards help to keep your motivation high.**

_____
_____
_____
_____
_____

Now let's talk more about keeping up motivation.

2. Improving Motivation to Discard

In the last class we talked about some ways to improve motivation to reduce clutter, and we discussed that it is normal for motivation to go up and down over time. In this chapter we will talk about another way to improve motivation, by using your imagination to see a clear room.

Visualize Your Decluttered Space

Another way to improve your motivation is to think about what each room in your home would look like if it was clear. Often this is difficult for people to do because it has been such a long time since the house was clear. So you will need to use your imagination.

As a class, close your eyes and imagine a certain room in your home being clear. Use as many of your senses as possible – what would the room look like, what would it smell like, where would the furniture be? Let's first practice as a class.

CLASS TASK: Using Your Imagination to Visualize Your Decluttered Space

Choose one room in your house and imagine that it is clear and tidy. How it is decorated? How does it smell? Where is the furniture placed in the room? Close your eyes and spend a few minutes imagining the room, then write down what it looks like below.

Visualization Worksheet: Example

Room: *My bedroom*

Describe the room as you would like it to be:

- *A clean bed with a clean floral comforter*
- *A bookshelf with books upright, not falling out and covered with dust*
- *Clean gray carpet*
- *A closet that is able to be closed*
- *No boxes or piles of clothes on the floor*
- *A chair that I can sit in*
- *A small table with space to put a cup of coffee and my glasses*
- *Walls nicely painted*
- *Room smells like lavender*

Visualization Worksheet

Item: _____

Room where it belongs: _____

Describe the room as you would like it to be:

_____

_____

_____

_____

_____

_____

_____

Now let's try something a little different. Let's practice using this image to help you discard. As you work through the item that you brought from home, answer the following questions.

1. When you picture the room as you would like it to be, does the item that you are considering holding on to fit in the picture?

YES / NO

2. Is keeping this item going to help you achieve the image that you see in your imagination?

YES / NO

3.   Being Motivated By Your Values

Next we are going to practice combining the skills from the last two classes as we practice discarding. Use the worksheet on the next page to help guide you. This was an example from one of our previous class members.

   The worksheet can also be used to help with your motivation when you want to acquire something.

Motivation Worksheet: Example

Item that I am considering discarding (or acquiring): *A beautiful blue decorative bowl*
Room in my home where it would be located: *Dining room*
When I visualize this room being clear, does the item belong there?   Yes / ⟨No⟩
What will be the advantages of discarding (or not acquiring) this item?

1.   *Reduce my clutter*
2.   *Help me to work towards being able to actually use my dining room table*

What are my "top 3" life goals and values?

1.   *Maintain good relationships with my kids and grandkids*
2.   *Take care of my health*
3.   *Get my finances in order*

Would discarding this item (or not acquiring this item) be consistent with these life goals and values?

If yes, can you discard (or not acquire) the item now?   ⟨Yes⟩ / No

If no, why are you saving this item?   Yes / ⟨No⟩
Because I will miss it …
Is this reason more important to you than the values you listed above? Yes / ⟨No⟩

If no, then please consider discarding the item (or not acquiring the item) and practice tolerating negative emotions that arise.

Motivation Worksheet

Item that I am considering discarding (or acquiring): _____
Room in my home where it would be located: _____
When I visualize this room being clear, does the item belong there?   Yes / No
What will be the advantages of discarding (or not acquiring) this item?

1. _____

2. _____

3. _____

   What are my "top 3" life goals and values?

1. _____

2. _____

3. _____

Would discarding (or not acquiring) this item be consistent with these life goals and values?
If yes, can you discard (or not acquire) the item now?   Yes / No
If no, why are you saving this item?   Yes / No

_____

_____

_____

Is this reason more important to you than the values you listed above?   Yes / No
If no, then please consider discarding the item (or not acquiring the item) and practice tolerating negative emotions that arise.

4.   Checking In on Long-Term SMART Goals

In Chapter 2 we spent some time setting a few short-term and long-term SMART goals. It is important to review these goals to make sure that you are on track to achieving them.

CLASS TASK: Checking In on Long-Term SMART goals

Look back to your long-term SMART goals (Chapter 2 of your workbook). Discuss as a group whether you are on track to achieving your long-term SMART goals. Make a plan around what you need to do to make sure that you achieve your SMART goals.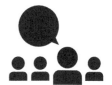

My Plan:

_____

_____

_____

_____

5.   Bad Guy Re-evaluation

CLASS TASK: Bad Guy Evaluation

Over the past two weeks we have talked about motivation. Take some time to evaluate how much you think this bad guy is contributing to your acquiring behavior and difficulty discarding over the past couple weeks. Rate from 0 (not a problem for me) to 10 (a very big problem for me).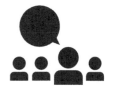

Acquiring: How much do you think low motivation is getting in the way of you resisting acquiring? In other words, are you feeling like you don't want to work on your clutter problem right now?

0 —— 1 —— 2 —— 3 —— 4 —— 5 —— 6 —— 7 —— 8 —— 9 —— 10

0 = Not a problem for me
10 = A very big problem for me

Discarding: How much do you think low motivation is getting in the way of you discarding? In other words, are you feeling unmotivated to work on your discarding right now? Or are you thinking that maybe your clutter isn't such a big problem after all?

0 —— 1 —— 2 —— 3 —— 4 —— 5 —— 6 —— 7 —— 8 —— 9 —— 10

0 = Not a problem for me
10 = A very big problem for me

How do your ratings today compare with your original ratings from Chapter 2?

If your score came down: Congratulations – you're beating the bad guy!

If your score remains the same (or is higher): We need to problem solve how you can practice the skills to beat this bad guy!

6.   Homework

Remember that people who do the most homework do the best at the end of the class. We recommend spending at least 1 hour a day working through your homework tasks.

Your homework this week is:

1.   **Reread information from week 10 (including Rita's story).**
2.   **Practice using the In and Out Log every day.**
3.   **Practice discarding for a minimum of 30 minutes per day.**
4.   **Complete weekly SMART goal.**
5.   **Bring lots of items from home to class next week.**
6.   **Other:** _____

My SMART goal for this week:
_____

What will be my personal reward for completing my SMART goal this week?
Reward: _____

When will I give myself the reward?
Day: _____

Did I accomplish my SMART goal?   Yes   No
If no, what got in the way? _____

Rita's Story

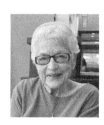

I hope that this lesson taught you some important skills for helping you to improve your motivation. I know that motivation is certainly something that I struggled with from time to time, both during the class and after the class ended.

If motivation is a problem for you then I would encourage you to practice these skills. It is important to remind yourself that it might take time to master these new skills!

It is almost time for you to start to put all the skills that you have learned in the class together and really work on your discarding. This is where I saw the most change in my clutter. I hope that you feel brave to really move forward with reducing your clutter too. I did it, so I'm sure you can too.

Rita.

In and Out Log – Week 10

Date	In	Out

Chapter 11/16

Putting It All Together

Part 1

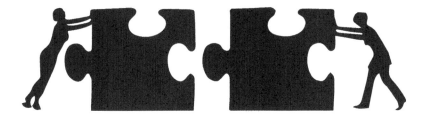

Overview

---

1. Homework Review

CLASS TASK: Homework Review

We will now go around the class and discuss each person's
homework and whether they have achieved their SMART goal.
  The homework tasks from last week were: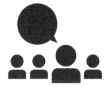

1. Reread information from week 10 (including Rita's story).
2. Practice using the In and Out Log every day.
3. Practice discarding for a minimum of 30 minutes per day.
4. Complete weekly SMART goal.
5. Bring lots of items from home to class next week.
6. Other: _____

- Did you accomplish your SMART goal for the week? If not, how will you change things to make it more likely you will succeed this week? **Remember that the more you practice the skills, the better you will be at the end of the class!**
- Did you reward yourself? **Remember that rewards help to keep your motivation high.**

_____

_____

_____

_____

_____

You have now learned about all the bad guys and how they contribute to your problem with clutter. You have also learned some practical techniques for addressing each of these bad guys. We hope that you are feeling more confident in your ability to overcome the bad guys, but learning a new skill takes a lot of practice.

For this reason, over the remaining weeks of the Declutter Class, we will get lots of practice using the skills that we have learned so far. It is very important that you bring in belongings from home *for every session*, because we will focus mainly on discarding over the remaining weeks. You will also need to bring a greater number of belongings than you have in the past classes.

In each of the "Putting it together" classes, we will also talk about some common barriers to discarding. These are problems that our other class members have discussed in the past.

Let's start by looking at these barriers.

2.   Troubleshooting Common Barriers

In addition to practicing discarding in each class from this point on, we will be introducing some solutions and strategies to deal with common problems that come up when decluttering.

Let's begin!

Barrier 1: Areas Getting Recluttered

"Even after I successfully declutter a particular area, it gets cluttered again – pretty quickly."

Even after you have successfully decluttered a target area, it's very easy to slip back into your old ways. In order to prevent this from happening, we recommend implementing a plan for regular upkeeping and strategies to maintain your motivation.

Regular upkeeping   It is helpful to make a plan in order to keep up with new items that come into your home (e.g., mail) and regular chores you have to do. By having a routine time of day for items such as mail, laundry, trash, etc., you will be better able to keep new clutter from developing. Here are some suggestions for routines for regular upkeeping.

- Pick a time to sort new mail and papers daily.
- Empty your trash twice per week (or more if needed).
- Take the trash out at the same time every week.
- Wash the dishes every day.
- Wash your clothes once a week (or more if needed).
- Set up a time and system for paying bills by the due date.
- Put away new items as soon as you bring them home, or at least that same day.

Let's come up with a plan for regular upkeeping for you. Write down your plan of how you will keep up with tasks such as mail, bills, dishes, laundry, and other incoming items. Are there other items for which you need to come up with a plan? Ask your fellow class members and class leaders for suggestions if needed.

   How I will keep up with:

Mail: _____

Bills: _____

Dishes: _____

Laundry: _____

Trash: _____

Other: _____

Other: _____

Other: _____

Barrier 2: Cannot Access the "Final Home" for Objects

"Where do I put things when its 'final home' is inaccessible? I am just churning."

This is a difficult challenge. As you learned previously, we want to minimize churning and the time it takes to make a decision about where to put an item. As much as possible, we want to make a decision once about whether to keep an item, where it belongs, and then put it there. But when you are in the beginning of your work on overcoming clutter, this can be hard to do, as the intended place for your item may already be cluttered with other items, and it's not possible to put the intended item there.

In these cases, we recommend you use an "intermediate staging area." This would be an area (or a box) where you put items that you have decided to keep, but the place where you intend to put the item is too cluttered right now or is inaccessible for some other reason.

Take a few minutes to think about areas in your home that are currently too cluttered and that you may have to use a staging area for until you declutter that area. We recommend creating the *least* amount of staging areas/boxes as possible.

Area in need of staging area	What I'll use as a staging area
Bedroom	Dining room

3.   Putting It All Together

Over the remaining weeks you will use a flowchart and practice the skills we have talked about previously to help you to discard. First choose an item from your box of belongings, then follow the flowchart. Over time we want you to be able to work through the flowchart very quickly.

We want you to try to discard as many items as possible. You will also discuss your progress with the other class members.

CLASS TASK: Putting the Skills Together

We now want you to practice discarding your belongings. Every now and then your class leaders will stop the class to discuss progress with the other class members.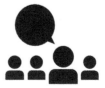

Use the flowchart to help make your decisions about what to do with the item, and also to determine which of the four "bad guys" is getting in the way. After you make a decision about one item, move onto the next. The goal is to discard as much as possible.

The only way to reduce the clutter in your home is to discard your items. **You can't have a clear house *and* all the belongings.**

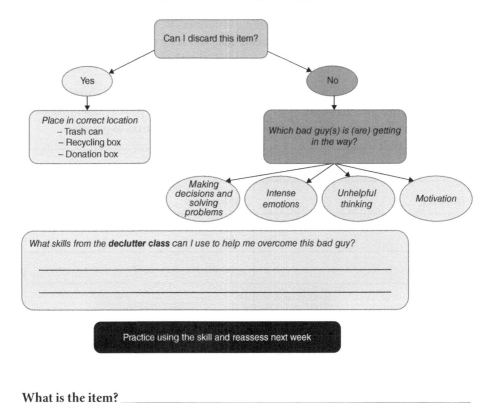

What is the item? _____

So now that you've practiced discarding while paying attention to the "bad guys," what did you learn?

Which of the bad guys still causes you the most problems with your discarding?

_____

_____

_____

_____

If you noticed that a certain "bad guy" keeps coming up, we recommend reviewing the appropriate chapters and practicing the skills described in them. For example, if intense emotions kept getting in the way, use the strategies introduced in Chapters 5 and 6 when attempting to discard.

4. Homework

Remember that people who do the most homework do the best at the end of the class. We recommend spending at least 1 hour a day working through your homework tasks.

Your homework this week is:

1. Reread information from week 11 (including Rita's story).
2. Practice using the In and Out Log every day.
3. Practice discarding for a minimum of 30 minutes per day.
4. Complete weekly SMART goal.
5. Bring lots of items from home to class next week.
6. Other: _____

My SMART goal for this week:
_____

What will be my personal reward for completing my SMART goal this week?
Reward: _____

When will I give myself the reward?
Day: _____

Did I accomplish my SMART goal?   Yes   No
If no, what got in the way? _____

Rita's Story

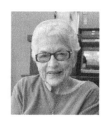

Congratulations on making it to the eleventh class! At this point, you have learned all the skills you need to tackle your clutter and acquiring problem. Now that you know all of the skills, it's really time to get down and apply them.

I found that learning or understanding a skill was not the same thing as applying it to help me overcome my clutter problem. Applying the skills is actually a lot harder! Knowing the skills won't do much for you unless you actually use them to help you discard or not acquire.

From this point on, you'll be spending the majority of your time in class actually practicing discarding – that is, applying the skills that you've learned so far. This is probably the most important part of the Declutter Class (and probably the most challenging). Let's face it, we're not going to make much progress with our clutter if we don't let go of things.

I wasn't sure how helpful it was going to be to focus on discarding in class. But I found that this part made the most difference in overcoming my clutter. Decluttering in class helped me to let go of things despite my fears of feeling regret later on. Discussing things with the class was particularly helpful for me – we were able to call each other out when we were avoiding discarding.

Good luck this week. Next week, you'll continue to practice discarding in class, as well as troubleshooting a few more common barriers to decluttering.

Rita.

In and Out Log – Week 11

Date	In	Out

Chapter 12/16

Putting It All Together

Part 2

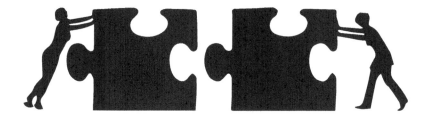

Overview

---

1. Homework Review

CLASS TASK: Homework Review

We will now go around the class and discuss each person's homework and whether they have achieved their SMART goal.
   The homework tasks from last week were:

1. **Reread information from week 11 (including Rita's story).**
2. **Practice using the In and Out Log every day.**
3. **Practice discarding for a minimum of 30 minutes per day.**
4. **Complete weekly SMART goal.**
5. **Bring lots of items from home to class next week.**
6. **Other: _____**

CBT for Hoarding Disorder: A Group Therapy Program Workbook, First Edition. David F. Tolin, Bethany M. Wootton, Blaise L. Worden, and Christina M. Gilliam.
© 2017 John Wiley & Sons Ltd. Published 2017 by John Wiley & Sons Ltd.

- Did you accomplish your SMART goal for the week? If not, how will you change things to make it more likely you will succeed this week? **Remember that the more you practice the skills, the better you will be at the end of the class!**
- Did you reward yourself? **Remember that rewards help to keep your motivation high.**

_____

_____

_____

_____

_____

2.   Troubleshooting Common Barriers

Just as we did in the last chapter, we will introduce two new common barriers that people in our previous classes have described.

Barrier 3: Conditions That Interfere with Discarding

"I have chronic pain or medical conditions that make it hard for me to practice discarding."

Sometimes people have other medical conditions that affect their mobility and make it difficult for them to practice sorting and discarding. However, at the same time, if you don't practice discarding, then your house won't become clear. So it is important to work out a way for you to still practice your discarding, but in a way that also allows you to manage your medical conditions. In our experience, the best way to do this is to pace the discarding.

In the Declutter Class we have emphasized discarding for 30 minutes a day, and this is the *minimum* that we recommend in order for class participants to make a significant dent in their clutter. However, this does not mean that it has to be 30 minutes all at once. Past class members have broken this up into more manageable time limits for them, such as two 15-minute internals or three 10-minute intervals. The point is that across the day your discarding adds up to *at least* 30 minutes a day. Of course, if you can do more than 30 minutes a day we highly encourage that.

So if you find that your medical conditions are getting in the way of your discarding, then it might be best to pace your discarding to a level that suits you. Remember, though, that discarding is an *essential* component of clearing your home, so it is important that you devote the time to it, but make the discarding time work for you.

If this barrier is a problem for you, what might be some ways you can work around this?

_____

_____

_____

_____

It might also be helpful for you to revisit the three steps of problem solving to help you deal with this problem:

- **Step 1:** *Name the problem*
- **Step 2:** *Brainstorm solutions and consider the pros and cons of each solution*
- **Step 3:** *Select preferred solution(s)*

Barrier 4: Not Having Information About What to Keep or Not Keep

"I feel like I am not sure what I really need to keep, or how long to keep it."

Even after working through the skills of the Declutter Class some people say they are still not sure what they should keep and what it is not necessary to keep. This is normal – often people want to be certain that they are not making a mistake about something. In this situation it might be helpful to go back and revisit some of the information that we talked about previously.

Chapter 8   In Chapter 8 we talked about some of the questions that can be helpful to ask yourself when you are thinking about discarding something. Some of the most important questions that apply to this situation include:

- **Would someone without a clutter problem keep the item?** If someone without a clutter problem would keep the item, then you may also need to keep it. This would include important documentation like birth certificates, passports, insurance information, and so on. However, if someone without a problem with clutter would throw it away, then you could also probably throw it away.
- **Would you be able to get the item again in the future if you needed it?** If you are able to get the item or information again in the future if you needed it, then you probably don't need to keep it and it can be discarded.
- **If you discarded the item, would something bad happen to you?** If there is a bad consequence of discarding the item, then you may need to keep it. A bad consequence might be something like losing your house or needing to pay a lot of money as a result. However, if the only negative consequence is one of intense emotions, then you can most likely discard the item because, as we learned in the Declutter Class, intense emotions will decline over time.

Chapter 3   In Chapter 3 we talked about guidelines for discarding. A lot of people find it helpful to go back and review these guidelines from time to time. In this situation some of the following rules may help:

- **The 12-month rule.** If you haven't used the item in the last 12 months, then chances are you are able to discard it.
- **The throw-it-away rule.** If your item is damaged in any way – stained, has holes in it, or is not working properly – then it is best just to throw it away.

In Chapter 3 we also talked about how much is too much to keep of any particular item. It might also be helpful to go back and revisit that part of your paperwork. It may help to answer the question about whether or not you need to keep the item.

If you have reviewed the Declutter Class materials and you are still unsure about whether or not you should throw the item away, then chances are you probably don't need to keep it and the item can be discarded. We understand that making the call on when to throw things away is difficult, but if you are not sure, then chances are you probably don't need it.

The good news is that over time you will find that making these decisions will become easier.

3.   Putting It All Together

Last week we practiced putting all the skills together and learned how to practice discarding using the discarding flowchart. In this class we will practice discarding again. Just like last week, you will stop your discarding and discuss your progress with the class from time to time.

We want you to practice discarding as many items as possible. Use the flowchart to assess each item and ask your class leader if you need help.

What is the item? _____

Can I discard this item?

Yes — Place in correct location
– Trash can
– Recycling box
– Donation box

No — Which bad guy(s) is (are) getting in the way?

- Making decisions and solving problems
- Intense emotions
- Unhelpful thinking
- Motivation

What skills from the **declutter class** can I use to help me overcome this bad guy?

_____

_____

Practice using the skill and reassess next week

4.   Homework

Remember that people who do the most homework do the best at the end of the class. We recommend spending at least 1 hour a day working through your homework tasks.

Your homework this week is:

1.   Reread information from week 12 (including Rita's story).
2.   Practice using the In and Out Log every day.
3.   Practice discarding for a minimum of 30 minutes per day.
4.   Complete weekly SMART goal.
5.   Bring lots of items from home to class next week.
6.   Other: _____

My SMART goal for this week:
_____

What will be my personal reward for completing my SMART goal this week?
Reward: _____

When will I give myself the reward?
Day: _____

Did I accomplish my SMART goal?   Yes   No
If no, what got in the way? _____

Rita's Story

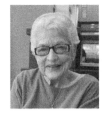

I hope you enjoyed the second "Putting it together" class and that you are using this time to really practice all the skills you have learned so far. I found that I was working through a lot more possessions in these classes, so it is helpful for you to brings lots of items to class.

I found the "Putting it together" classes to be really helpful and I think this is where I made the most progress with clearing my house. I know it is not easy, but for me steady progress was really the key. Plus spending the time in class discarding meant that I was getting through even more clutter than I normally would at home.

I also liked helping the other people in the class to discard. It made me proud that we were all doing so well and making big changes in our lives. Other class members really challenged me, and although it was difficult, I think it helped me (and them) in the end.

The problems for troubleshooting that we talked about in the class this week didn't really apply to me, but other people in the class found the information to be really useful. Even though we have covered some of the information before, I think it can be helpful to be reminded about things because, after all, we learned a lot of information really quickly over the past few months.

Good luck with your discarding this week. I hope that you reach your SMART goal this week too.

Rita.

In and Out Log – Week 12

Date	In	Out

Chapter 13/16

Putting It All Together

Part 3

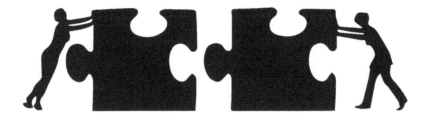

1.   Homework Review

CLASS TASK: Homework Review

We will now go around the class and discuss each person's homework and whether they have achieved their SMART goal.
The homework tasks from last week were:

1.   **Reread information from week 12 (including Rita's story).**
2.   **Practice using the In and Out Log every day.**
3.   **Practice discarding for a minimum of 30 minutes per day.**
4.   **Complete weekly SMART goal.**
5.   **Bring lots of items from home to class next week.**
6.   **Other:** _____

CBT for Hoarding Disorder: A Group Therapy Program Workbook, First Edition. David F. Tolin,
Bethany M. Wootton, Blaise L. Worden, and Christina M. Gilliam.
© 2017 John Wiley & Sons Ltd. Published 2017 by John Wiley & Sons Ltd.

- Did you accomplish your SMART goal for the week? If not, how will you change things to make it more likely you will succeed this week? **Remember that the more you practice the skills, the better you will be at the end of the class!**
- Did you reward yourself? **Remember that rewards help to keep your motivation high.**

_____

_____

_____

_____

_____

_____

2.   Troubleshooting Common Barriers

As we have done in the previous weeks, we will also discuss solutions and strategies to deal with common problems that can come up when people are decluttering.

Barrier 5: My Family Member Also Has Hoarding Disorder

"I am having a hard time decluttering because many items aren't mine, and my family member isn't helping maintain the areas I've already decluttered."

As we discussed earlier in the Declutter Class, hoarding has a strong genetic influence. This means that often we find that family members of our class members also often have problems with clutter. Sometimes the family member is aware of the problem and wants to address it, but sometimes they do not want to change their behavior.

If the family member *does* want to address their problem, then it might be helpful for them to enroll in a class like the Declutter Class where they will learn skills to help them discard and reduce the clutter in their home. We don't recommend that family members take part in the same class at the same time, however, because it may negatively impact the class dynamics and may lead to a less favorable outcome for the family members. We also don't recommend that you try to teach your family member the skills because you are only new to learning them yourself. It is important that they attend a class that is delivered by trained class leaders.

Other times the family member does not want to change. This can be a tricky situation for our class members because they are working hard to clear parts of the home while their family member does not want them to discard items or fills the home up with other items. Remember that you can only change yourself. There is no point getting into never-ending arguments about clutter. However, this is a good opportunity to be a good role model for your loved one! Show them how discarding and decluttering is beneficial and easier than expected.

Barrier 6: I Feel Like I Can't Get Rid of Items If They Are Worth Money

Often people have difficulty discarding because they feel like they cannot discard anything if it is worth any amount of money, even a very small amount. Often this leads people to want to sell the item rather than discarding it. This makes sense because often people with a problem with clutter do not want to be wasteful. However, selling the item often takes a lot more planning and effort than just discarding it.

Because people with hoarding disorder often have trouble with planning and following through with their plans, we recommend that people discard most items and try to sell very few. We find that often when people try to sell the item they just end up keeping it because it is too much effort. This means that it takes a lot longer to clear out your home.

If this is a barrier that you find yourself coming up against, then it might be helpful to make some deadlines for yourself. For instance, "If I don't sell the item within two weeks, then I must discard it by throwing it in the trash or donating it to charity."

Work through the following questions to help you make deadlines about items that you want to sell.

What are some items in your home that you are reluctant to discard because you believe they are worth money?

1. _____
2. _____
3. _____
4. _____
5. _____

How can you sell these items quickly?

1. _____
2. _____
3. _____
4. _____
5. _____

What is a reasonable deadline to sell the items within (e.g., 1 week or 2 weeks)?

1. _____
2. _____
3. _____
4. _____
5. _____

How will you discard the items if you do not sell them by the deadline?

1. _____

2. _____

3. _____

4. _____

5. _____

3.   Putting It All Together

For the last few weeks we practiced putting all the skills together and learned how to practice discarding using the discarding flowchart. We know that when we are learning any new behavior we have to practice a lot before we get really good at it. This is the point of the remaining classes. We want you to practice discarding over and over so that you become very good at making decisions about discarding.

In the class this week we will practice discarding again, and from time to time we will stop and review your progress. Use the flowchart (if you need to) to assess each item and ask your class leader if you need help.

What is the item?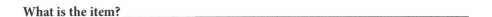

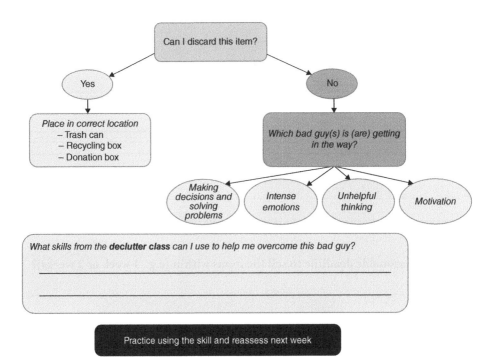

4.   Homework

Remember that people who do the most homework do the best at the end of the class. We recommend spending at least 1 hour a day working through your homework tasks.

Your homework this week is:

1.   Reread information from week 13 (including Rita's story).
2.   Practice using the In and Out Log every day.
3.   Practice discarding for a minimum of 30 minutes per day.
4.   Complete weekly SMART goal.
5.   Bring lots of items from home to class next week.
6.   Other: _____

My SMART goal for this week:
_____

What will be my personal reward for completing my SMART goal this week?
Reward: _____

When will I give myself the reward?
Day: _____

Did I accomplish my SMART goal?   Yes   No
If no, what got in the way? _____

Rita's Story

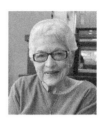

Hi everyone. Good work for making it this far through the class. I know from my own experience that it hasn't been easy, and a few members in my class didn't make it this far!

In the class this week you got to practice a lot more with discarding and you also learned about some more common barriers for people who have problems with clutter. I was able to relate to both of the obstacles this week and I found discussing these barriers as a class really helpful. I wasn't alone when it came to these problems. A lot of people in the class could identify with them as well. We were able to make a plan about how to address the barriers over the remaining weeks of the class.

As always, I found it helpful (but challenging) to practice discarding as well. I noticed that I felt like I was starting to get better at discarding. I was able to make decisions about different items faster and I felt less of the negative emotions when I was discarding. I knew I still had a long way to go, but it felt good to see some progress too. I was proud of the other class members as well. You could see that we were all really trying hard.

Good luck this week.
Rita.

In and Out Log – Week 13

Date	In	Out

Chapter 14/16

Putting It All Together

Part 4

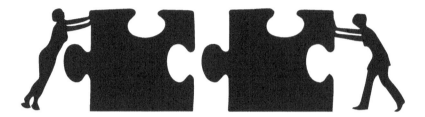

Overview

---

1.   Homework Review

CLASS TASK: Homework Review

We will now go around the class and discuss each person's homework and whether they have achieved their SMART goal.

The homework tasks from last week were:

1. **Reread information from week 13 (including Rita's story).**
2. **Practice using the In and Out Log every day.**
3. **Practice discarding for a minimum of 30 minutes per day.**
4. **Complete weekly SMART goal.**
5. **Bring lots of items from home to class next week.**
6. **Other:** _____

CBT for Hoarding Disorder: A Group Therapy Program Workbook, First Edition. David F. Tolin,
Bethany M. Wootton, Blaise L. Worden, and Christina M. Gilliam.
© 2017 John Wiley & Sons Ltd. Published 2017 by John Wiley & Sons Ltd.

- Did you accomplish your SMART goal for the week? If not, how will you change things to make it more likely you will succeed this week? **Remember that the more you practice the skills, the better you will be at the end of the class!**
- Did you reward yourself? **Remember that rewards help to keep your motivation high.**

_____

_____

_____

_____

_____

2. Troubleshooting Common Barriers

As we have done in the previous weeks, we will also discuss solutions and strategies to deal with common problems that can come up when people are decluttering. This week we will address one common barrier. We also want you to come up with another barrier that you have been experiencing and discuss as a class how you can overcome this barrier.

Barrier 7: Being Overly Careful When Discarding

"I can discard things, but first I have to do a lot of time-consuming preparation."

This is a common barrier that often comes up for people in our class. Often what happens is they discard things, but first they have to do a lot of time-consuming activities such as calling others to see if they want the item, shredding every piece of paper, making sure things go in the correct recycling bin or that they go to charity rather than in the trash. Often when people face this barrier they have very rigid rules around how to discard items and they don't like to do it any other way.

A key message from the Declutter Class is to discard things quickly and to clear your home as much as possible within a short period of time. Obviously if discarding a single item takes a lot of time, then you won't get your house as decluttered as you would like.

If this is a barrier for you, we recommend practicing discarding things the "wrong" way. This means discarding things without following your strict rules. For instance, discarding the item without calling others to check if they want it, or throwing away paper in the trash without shredding it first. This will allow you to discard much faster and get through more items in your sorting and discarding sessions. This will ultimately mean a clear house much faster.

This is not an easy thing to do, but with practice it will become easier and you will see that you are clearing more items in your home.

What are some of the rules that you have about discarding that might be getting in the way of discarding?

_____

_____

_____

Additional Barriers (Optional)

Barrier 8:

_____

_____

_____

_____

_____

Techniques/solutions:

_____

_____

_____

_____

_____

_____

3.   Putting It All Together

For the last few weeks we practiced putting all the skills together and learned how to practice discarding using the discarding flowchart. We know that when we are learning any new behavior we have to practice a lot before we get really good at it. We want you to practice discarding over and over so that you become very good at making decisions about discarding. Hopefully you will notice some improvements in your ability to make decisions when discarding and that you are able to discard much faster than you could previously.

Let's spend more time practicing.

What is the item? _____

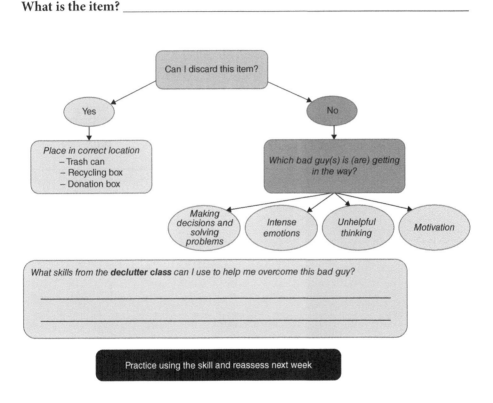

4.   Homework

Remember that people who do the most homework do the best at the end of the class. We recommend spending at least 1 hour a day working through your homework tasks.

Your homework this week is:

1. Reread information from week 14 (including Rita's story).
2. Practice using the In and Out Log every day.
3. Practice discarding for a minimum of 30 minutes per day.
4. Complete weekly SMART goal.
5. Bring lots of items from home to class next week.
6. Other: _____

My SMART goal for this week:
_____

What will be my personal reward for completing my SMART goal this week?
Reward: _____

When will I give myself the reward?
Day: _____

Did I accomplish my SMART goal?   Yes   No
If no, what got in the way? _____

Rita's Story

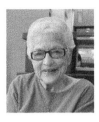

Hi everyone. You have almost made it the whole way through the Declutter Class. Congratulations!

In the class this week my class members and I practiced more discarding (because practice makes perfect, right?). I was so proud of all the progress that we had all made (and will continue to make). I know it hasn't been easy for people and it hasn't been easy for me either, but most of us were making such good progress.

In the class this week you got to practice a lot more with discarding and you also learned about some more common barriers for people who have problems with clutter. I was able to relate to the obstacle again this week and I found that discussing the "rules" that I had for discarding as a class was really helpful. We all seemed to have different rules about how things should be discarded. I could see that having these strict rules really impacts how much clutter I get through when I am discarding.

We also discussed another barrier that one of the class members raised in the class, and that was how do we continue to improve after the class ends? I have been feeling sad that the class will be ending soon and a little worried about whether I will be able to keep up the good progress that I had made, so it seems that this was a common theme across a lot of class members.

We discussed this as a class and came up with some good solutions. Our class leaders also told us that we would learn more about this in the next class.

Good luck this week.
Rita.

In and Out Log – Week 14

Date	In	Out

Chapter 15/16

Staying Clutter Free in the Future
Part 1

1. Homework Review

CLASS TASK: Homework Review

We will now go around the class and discuss each person's homework and whether they have achieved their SMART goal.
The homework tasks from last week were:

1. **Reread information from week 14 (including Rita's story).**
2. **Practice using the In and Out Log every day.**
3. **Practice discarding for a minimum of 30 minutes per day.**

CBT for Hoarding Disorder: A Group Therapy Program Workbook, First Edition. David F. Tolin,
Bethany M. Wootton, Blaise L. Worden, and Christina M. Gilliam.
© 2017 John Wiley & Sons Ltd. Published 2017 by John Wiley & Sons Ltd.

4. **Complete weekly SMART goal.**
5. **Bring lots of items from home to class next week.**
6. **Other:** _____

- Did you accomplish your SMART goal for the week? If not, how will you change things to make it more likely you will succeed this week? **Remember that the more you practice the skills, the better you will be at the end of the class!**
- Did you reward yourself? **Remember that rewards help to keep your motivation high.**

_____

_____

_____

_____

_____

2.   Reviewing Progress

What You've Learned

Now you know how to recognize and fight all the bad guys that contribute to your hoarding behaviors. Below is a reminder list of some of the main things you've learned. As we review the list, check off the ones that you think have been the most helpful.

1. *Making efficient decisions and solving problems effectively*
    - Use the problem-solving model: Brainstorm possible solutions without judging. Try the solution(s) and evaluate the results.
    - Use the 10 guidelines for discarding and stopping acquiring.
    - Schedule times for discarding.
    - Improve organization by having a home for every category of items.
    - Know and avoid high-risk situations.

2. *Not so intense emotions*
    - Notice your emotions and describe/accept them; you don't need to let them be the boss.
    - "Ride the wave": All strong emotions will decrease with time if you let them.

3. *More helpful thinking*
    - Question the thoughts: Rather than accepting your thoughts, question them. Are they helpful or unhelpful?
    - Act as you would advise a friend: Respond to situations as you would advise a friend, rather than just accepting your thoughts as truth.

4. *Maintaining strong motivation*
   - Increase your motivation by writing down the costs and benefits of discarding, or the costs and benefits of acquiring.
   - Maintain motivation by setting realistic, concrete goals and making sure that you reward yourself after you accomplish your goal.
   - Focus on your goals and values to help you to resist acquiring and increase your discarding.
   - Use your imagination to help you see a house that is clutter free.

What are the top 3 skills from the Declutter Class that you have found to be the most helpful?

1. _____

2. _____

3. _____

Choosing How You Think About Progress

Remember that progress takes time. You did not acquire all of your items overnight! It was likely a gradual process over many years. Decluttering is often that way, too. By completing this program, you are all well on your way to achieving your goals of having a clear home, but it is unlikely that your house will be completely clear by the end of the class!

Oftentimes, we hear class members having mixed reactions to their progress, such as "Well, that's good progress, but I still have so much to do!" Or possibly more negative thoughts such as "I didn't achieve as much as I hoped."

CLASS TASK: Write Down Your Thoughts About Your Progress

_____

_____

_____

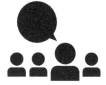

Remember that our thoughts influence how we feel, and how we behave! And remember that our thoughts are not necessarily true. Share your thoughts with the class. Are they accurate? Might they influence how you behave? Would you judge another class member as harshly?

When we feel overly pessimistic about our progress and don't give ourselves credit for the hard work that we do, it is even more difficult to keep up the hard work that decluttering takes. Remember to celebrate your successes, and to focus on what you have done, not just what is left to do.

Keep in mind that you have total control over how much progress you make from here on out: Now you have the skills, so keep practicing them so they become more and more automatic.

3.   Practice Discarding

Earlier in the class you identified the aspects of the class that you found the most helpful. While this is important, it is also helpful to identify those skills that you still need more practice with. What are the aspects of the class that you think you need to practice more in order to achieve your goals? This might be using the skills to address one of the bad guys, or it might just be more practice discarding.

1. _____

2. _____

3. _____

CLASS TASK: Discarding Practice

For the rest of the class practice discarding, identifying one skill or bad guy that you need more practice with. Discuss with the class what you need to do to improve this skill and spend some time practicing this skill over the next week.

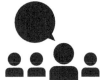

4.   Homework

Remember that people who do the most homework do the best at the end of the class. We recommend spending at least 1 hour a day working through your homework tasks.

Your homework this week is:

1. **Reread information from week 15 (including Rita's story).**
2. **Practice using the In and Out Log every day.**
3. **Practice discarding for a minimum of 30 minutes per day.**
4. **Complete weekly SMART goal.**
5. **Other:** _____

My SMART goal for this week:

_____

What will be my personal reward for completing my SMART goal this week?
Reward: _____

When will I give myself the reward?
Day: _____

Did I accomplish my SMART goal?   Yes   No
If no, what got in the way? _____

Rita's Story

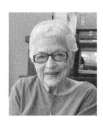

Hi everyone. You have almost made it the whole way through the Declutter Class. Well done! I hope that you are proud of yourself!

This week you started to focus on wrapping up the class.

In the class this week I really had time reflecting on how far I had come. I guess I didn't realize just how much I had discarded over the last 15 weeks. I felt proud of myself (and the other class members), but at the same time it was good to catch the unhelpful thinking that might get in the way of me progressing further.

I could recognize thoughts like "I'll never be able to continue on my own" and "I should have cleared more stuff than this." I know that when I think this way it really affects my mood – I feel scared and sad. So I know I need to make sure that my thinking is more realistic and that I don't let myself dwell on thoughts like this.

In this class I felt like I needed more practice with tackling the intense emotions bad guy. I know this is a real problem for me and I know that I need to work more on this. In class I practiced discarding some difficult items and watched my emotions gradually decline. It was scary for me, but it is good to see that the emotion does decrease on its own. I practiced this a lot over the next week.

Good luck to you this week. Next week is the final class!

Rita.

In and Out Log – Week 15

Date	In	Out

Chapter 16/16

Staying Clutter Free in the Future
Part 2

1.   Homework Review

CLASS TASK: Homework Review

We will now go around the class and discuss each person's homework and whether they have achieved their SMART goal.
  The homework tasks from last week were:

1.   **Reread information from week 15 (including Rita's story).**
2.   **Practice using the In and Out Log every day.**
3.   **Practice discarding for a minimum of 30 minutes per day.**
4.   **Complete weekly SMART goal.**
5.   **Other:** _____

CBT for Hoarding Disorder: A Group Therapy Program Workbook, First Edition. David F. Tolin,
Bethany M. Wootton, Blaise L. Worden, and Christina M. Gilliam.
© 2017 John Wiley & Sons Ltd. Published 2017 by John Wiley & Sons Ltd.

- Did you accomplish your SMART goal for the week? If not, how will you change things to make it more likely you will succeed this week? **Remember that the more you practice the skills, the easier it will be to continue discarding after the class ends!**

- Did you reward yourself? **Remember that rewards help to keep your motivation high.**

_____

_____

_____

_____

_____

2.   Maintaining Motivation

Overcoming hoarding is hard work and it takes time (usually longer than the 16-week Declutter Class). In order to make progress on your hoarding problem, it's important that you find ways to sustain your motivation. Here are some suggestions from past participants in our class:

1.   **Reward yourself.**   One way to keep your motivation up is to make sure that you are rewarding yourself for your efforts and your successes. Reward yourself each time you *complete* a sorting session – the amount of time you set out to sort. These rewards don't have to be time consuming or costly. Think about what kind of things you would find rewarding, and write them down on the following page. Make sure that you reward yourself after each sorting session, but not until you actually sort for the designated amount of time or clear the particular area.

2.   **Be patient with yourself.**   Remember that overcoming hoarding is hard work, and changes are not going to happen overnight. For many people who begin sorting/discarding, the clutter may actually appear to worsen in the beginning. Remember that the goal of sorting/discarding is NOT to do things perfectly. It's OK if you're not 100% sure where to put a particular item. Just pick the best choice possible in that moment, and move on. You can always come back to things later and change them, if you really need to. Also remember that sorting and discarding will get easier with practice – that is, the more you practice sorting, the better you will become about making decisions (keep, let go, choose category and location). You will also find that the more you practice sorting and discarding, the less distressing the task will become.

3.   **Use the skills you've learned so far.**   If you're feeling less motivated, go back to the Motivation chapters and practice the skills that we discussed. Also review the goals you set out at the beginning of the class (week 2) and revisit your goals and values.

My Rewards for Working on My Hoarding Problem

Write down some goals and rewards for yourself. This strategy can be particularly helpful if you are feeling unmotivated or struggling to get started on a project.

Remember to pick goals that are specific, concrete, and realistic!

Goal setting example

Goal for today: *Sort through paperwork on top of kitchen table for one hour*

After I accomplish this goal, I will reward myself with: *Watch my favorite TV show – guilt free!*

CLASS TASK: Identify Some Goals and Rewards

Identify some goals and rewards for yourself below. Include some short-term goals (over the next week) and some long-term goals (to achieve over the next few months to years). Often long-term goals are bigger goals (which should also attract bigger rewards)!

Short-term goals:

1. Date: _____
Goal: _____

After I accomplish this goal, I will reward myself by/with:

_____

2. Date: _____
Goal: _____

After I accomplish this goal, I will reward myself by/with:

_____

Long-term goals:

1. Date: _____
Goal: _____

After I accomplish this goal, I will reward myself by/with:

_____

2. Date: _____
Goal: _____

After I accomplish this goal, I will reward myself by/with:

_____

3.   Wrap-Up and Questions

Congratulations on completing the Declutter Class! You have put a lot of effort into getting to this point, and we hope that your progress will continue over the coming weeks and months.

We encourage you all to stay in touch with each other after completion of the class. We have found that past class members sometimes like to share information and talk or get together after the end of the class. If you wish to do so, that is OK with us. If you do not wish to do this, that is OK too.

Please ask your class leaders if you have any final questions or concerns. Congratulations again on all of your hard work! You now have all of the skills you need to successfully declutter. Keep it up!

Great job!

Rita's Story

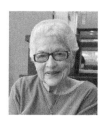

Hi everyone. Congratulations on getting the whole way through the Declutter Class. You should be really proud of yourself, because I know that it wasn't easy!

I hope that over the past 16 weeks you have learned some useful skills for reducing your clutter, but the most important part is actually practicing the skills. I made a deal with myself that I would review the class materials at the same time that I would normally come to the Declutter Class.

The people in my class exchanged contact details and from time to time some of us meet up for a coffee. I noticed that people made different levels of progress after the class ended. Some people did well and others did not do well at all. I found that continuing to practice the skills and setting SMART goals for myself each week after the course ended really helped me to continue to progress, and I would encourage you to do the same. It certainly wasn't all smooth sailing. I had periods of time where I did not discard anything for several days. I felt really down on myself and wanted to give up. But I reviewed the information (especially the motivation section) and I was able to keep going.

It has now been almost 12 months since I finished the Declutter Class and the bulk of my clutter is gone! I can see areas of my home that I have not been able to access for a VERY long time. It is such a great feeling! I know that you will also get there – as long as you keep practicing the skills! It is true what they say – the more you practice, the easier it is to make decisions about things, and the less distress it causes to throw things away.

That's it from me. I know that everyone is different, but I hope that you have learned something from my experience (and my mistakes).

I wish you all the best for the future.

Rita.

Reward Monitoring Sheet

Week	*Homework complete?*
Week 1	○ Yes ○ No
Week 2	○ Yes ○ No
Week 3	○ Yes ○ No
Week 4	○ Yes ○ No
Week 5	○ Yes ○ No
Week 6	○ Yes ○ No
Week 7	○ Yes ○ No
Week 8	○ Yes ○ No
Week 9	○ Yes ○ No
Week 10	○ Yes ○ No
Week 11	○ Yes ○ No
Week 12	○ Yes ○ No
Week 13	○ Yes ○ No
Week 14	○ Yes ○ No
Week 15	○ Yes ○ No
Week 16	○ Yes ○ No

Index

CBT for Hoarding Disorder: A Group Therapy Program Workbook, First Edition. David F. Tolin, Bethany M. Wootton, Blaise L. Worden, and Christina M. Gilliam.
© 2017 John Wiley & Sons Ltd. Published 2017 by John Wiley & Sons Ltd.

Printed and bound by CPI Group (UK) Ltd, Croydon, CR0 4YY

27/10/2024

14580362-0005